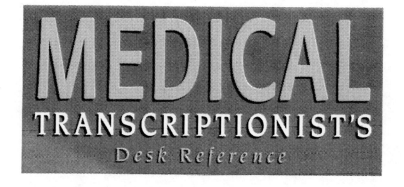

MEDICAL TRANSCRIPTIONIST'S *Desk Reference*

MEDICAL
TRANSCRIPTIONIST'S
Desk Reference

Carolyn Collins-Gates

SAUNDERS

An Imprint of Elsevier

SAUNDERS
An Imprint of Elsevier

11830 Westline Industrial Drive
St. Louis, Missouri 63146

Medical Transcriptionist's Desk Reference

NOTICE

Allied Health is an ever-changing field. Standard safety precautions must be followed, but as new research and clinical experience broaden our knowledge, changes in treatment and drug therapy may become necessary or appropriate. Readers are advised to check the most current product information provided by the manufacturer of each drug to be administered to verify the recommended dose, the method and duration of administration, and contraindications. It is the responsibility of the licensed prescriber, relying on experience and knowledge of the patient, to determine dosages and the best treatment for each individual patient. Neither the publisher nor the author assumes any liability for any injury and/or damage to persons or property arising from this publication.

Every attempt has been made to provide information that is accurate and consistent with current practice. However, errors can occur, and the reader is cautioned that neither the author nor the publisher assumes any responsibility for the reader's use of this material or for any damages resulting from the reader's use.

ISBN-13: 978-0-7216-9763-5
ISBN-10: 0-7216-9763-1

Acquisitions Editor: Susan Cole
Project Manager: Joy Moore
Designer: Amy Buxton

Printed in the United States of America

Last digit is the print number: 9 8 7

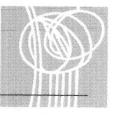

About the Author

Carolyn Collins-Gates has been contributing to the field of medical transcription for 35 years. She has worked as a medical transcriptionist, developed and taught course curricula in medical transcription, and devoted more than 20 years to providing medical transcription services in South Carolina.

Certified by the American Association for Medical Transcription (AAMT) in 1983, Ms. Collins-Gates is the founder and past President of the South Carolina Chapter of the AAMT. She currently serves as the Program Coordinator of the Midlands Chapter and Vice President of CRAAMT (North Carolina/South Carolina Regional Chapter).

Ms. Collins-Gates presently holds a position as instructor and program coordinator for basic and advanced medical transcription at Midlands Technical College; manages the transcription department at Lexington Medical Center; and serves as Vice President, Partner, and Consultant of Emergency Medicine Transcription Service of South Carolina, Inc.

To my children, Angie, Lori, Austin;
to my mother, Dorothy Q. Collins;
and to my brother, Ronald L. Collins, MD,
for all their love, support and encouragement.

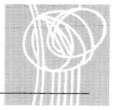

Preface

Welcome to *The Medical Transcriptionist's Desk Reference*. This handy reference tool is the one students, "newbies," and experienced medical transcriptionists alike reach for first to find answers quickly and easily.

Unique features include the following:

- **Just the Right Amount of Content**

Learning where to find resource information can be confusing, especially for students and new professionals. Valuable time is wasted searching through resources with too much detail. The simpler scope of this reference tool makes it easy to find answers to questions that arise every day, and the information is relevant because this book is written with direct reference to the style guidelines of the American Association for Medical Transcription (AAMT).

- **Intuitive Organization**

The topics in this reference are organized not as a medical doctor would by specialty but as the medical transcriptionist would by type of problem or situation most often encountered. Categories include sample reports and letters, medical terminology, terms related to physical examinations, and other lists of useful information; for example, lab tests, medications, and commonly confused words.

- **Quick Find Presentation**

Time is money for the medical transcriptionist. A quick scan down the contents in the front of the book provides a page number for each major topic covered. Easy-to-read lists make it easy to pinpoint information.

The Medical Transcriptionist's Desk Reference takes a unique and more effective approach to helping students and practicing medical transcriptionists make the most of their time and resources by providing a trusted reference tool that's easy to use.

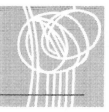

Acknowledgments

Sincere appreciation is given to Lexington Medical Center, Pamela Landers-Helms, BA, MT; Shirley Hilton, MT, ASCP; Betty Lewis, MT; Freida McCorkle, RT; Juliana Ott, ASCP, SM; Wynee Rich, BSH, RT (R)(T); Carol Rikard, RHIA, CTR; Jeannie Stevens, CST, RRT, RCP; Jeannie Thomas, BA, MT; Fred Vallejo, PT, MS; and Cathy Wendell, RHIA. They have all given their time, energy, and resources to the publication of this material.

The publisher would also like to thank the following reviewers:

Sharon B. Allred, BRE, CMT
Instructor
Guilford Technical Community College
Jamestown, North Carolina

Celeste Harjehausen, BS
Director of Client Services
Career Step, LLC
Springville, Utah

Melissa LaCour, RHIA
Program Director and Assistant Professor of Health Information Technology
Delgado Community College
New Orleans, Louisiana

Mary E. Seese, CMT
Certified Medical Transcriptionist
Huntersville, North Carolina

Susan Steinriede, EdD
Chair, Office Information Technology Department
Trident Technical College
Charleston, South Carolina

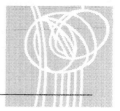

Contents

C H A P T E R 1

MEDICAL TRANSCRIPTION FORMATTING *1*

Style Guidelines *1*
Sample Medical Reports *4*
Sample Medical Letters *25*
Microsoft Word Keyboard Shortcuts *27*

C H A P T E R 2

MEDICAL TERMINOLOGY *29*

Prefixes and Suffixes *29*
Combining Forms *31*
Commonly Used Medical Terms *32*

C H A P T E R 3

PHYSICAL EXAMINATION TERMS *35*

General Terms *35*
Terms Related to Vital Signs *37*
Terms Related to the Skin *37*
Terms Related to HEENT *38*
Terms Related to the Neck *44*
Terms Related to the Chest and Breasts *45*
Terms Related to the Lungs *46*
Terms Related to the Heart *48*
Terms Related to the Abdomen *49*
Terms Related to the Back *51*
Terms Related to the Extremities *52*

Terms Related to the Rectum *55*
Terms Related to the Genitourinary Tract and Pelvis *56*
Terms Related to Neurological Conditions *58*
Terms Related to Mental Status *61*

C H A P T E R 4

BODY SYSTEMS *63*

Cardiovascular System *63*
Digestive System *69*
Endocrine System *72*
Integumentary System *73*
Musculoskeletal System *74*
Nervous System and Psychiatry *78*
Reproductive System *81*
Respiratory System *83*
Urinary System *85*

C H A P T E R 5

ONCOLOGY *89*

Cancer Classifications *89*
Radiation Oncology Terms *90*
Oncology Medications *92*

C H A P T E R 6

LABORATORY TESTS *103*

Medicare Chemistry Panels *103*
Complete Blood Count with Differential *103*

Normal Laboratory Values   *104*
Laboratory Tests   *105*
Laboratory Test Abbreviations   *111*

C H A P T E R 7

MICROBIOLOGY   *117*

Gram-Positive Aerobic Bacteria   *117*
Gram-Negative Aerobic Bacteria   *119*
Yeast and Yeast-like Microorganisms   *123*
Anaerobes   *125*
Haemophilus   *127*

C H A P T E R 8

RADIOLOGY   *129*

Radiology Studies   *129*

C H A P T E R 9

DRUG LISTS   *139*

Commonly Used Drugs   *139*
Commonly Confused Drug Names   *159*

C H A P T E R 10

CONFUSING WORDS, ABBREVIATIONS, AND EPONYMS   *163*

Commonly Misused Words   *163*
Commonly Used Medical Abbreviations   *170*
American and International Symbols, Abbreviations, and Measurements   *178*
Medical Credentials   *179*
Commonly Used Eponyms   *187*

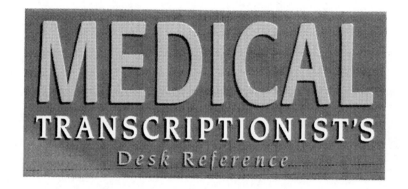

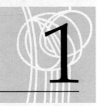

Medical Transcription Formatting

STYLE GUIDELINES

1. Always type the headings in bold uppercase letters, followed by a colon, if the text follows on the same line; for example, **REVIEW OF SYSTEMS:** If the heading appears on a separate line from the text, no colon is included after the heading.

2. Single-space all reports and double-space between paragraphs.

3. In the body of a report, dates should be written out; for example, January 1, 2002. All dates in the header of a legal record should be 8 digits; for example, 01/01/2002.

4. Use numerals (even if under 10) when typing weight, height, measurements, age, lab data, or technical expressions; however, do not begin a sentence with a numeral.

5. Dictated: "0", double "0", or triple "0" suture. Type: 0, 2-0, or 3-0 suture.

6. A colon should be used when typing a ratio. Dictated: Cardiothoracic ratio is 25 over 80. Type: Cardiothoracic ratio 25:80.

7. A slash (/) should be used to indicate "over" in dictation with blood pressures or chemical measurements. Dictated: Blood pressure 140 over 80. Type: Blood pressure 140/80.

8. A slash (/) is used to separate numbers indicating visual acuity. Dictated: Visual acuity twenty twenty. Type: Visual acuity 20/20.

9. A slash (/) is used for "per." Dictated: Pulse 80 per minute. Cholesterol is 390 mg/dl. Type: Pulse 80/minute, cholesterol 390 mg/dl. Dictated: Urinalysis reveals twenty red blood cells per high-powered field. Type: Urinalysis reveals 20 RBCs/hpf.

10. Do not use contractions unless they are part of a direct quote. Dictated: can't, won't, etc. Type: cannot, will not, etc.

11. Units of measure should always be typed on the same line; for example, with "4 mm," the 4 should be on the next line with unit of measure when possible.

12. Do not use an apostrophe with plural uppercase abbreviations; for example, WBCs, RBCs.

13. Do not type periods with credentials; for example, RN, MD, DO, PA.

14. When typing medications, do not type BID, TID, etc. Type b.i.d., t.i.d., q.i.d., q.4h., q.o.d., q.p.m., q.a.m., etc. Using the uppercased letters emphasizes the dosage more than the medication.

15. Do not type an additional period at the end of a sentence if an abbreviation is used at the end of a sentence; for example, Darvocet N 100 b.i.d.

16. Do not type an apostrophe with age. Dictated: Patient is in her forties. Type: Patient is in her 40s.

17. Uppercase all allergies/reactions; for example, ALLERGIES: PENICILLIN CAUSES A RASH. If the patient has no allergies, type ALLERGIES: None known.

18. Spell out American measurements but abbreviate international measurements without periods; for example, weight, height, inches, feet, quart, cc, mm, mg, dl, L, G, etc.

19. Uppercase all letters of most acronyms; however, do not uppercase the spelled out version unless it is a proper name.

    VBAC—vaginal birth after cesarean

    AMA—American Medical Association

20. Capitalize race, not color. Do not change white to Caucasian or black to African American. Type what the physician dictates.

21. Capitalize formal names of diseases and bacteria; for example, Crohn, Alzheimer.

22. Capitalize brand-name drugs but not generic drugs; for example, Tegretol and carbamazepine.

23. Use nonpossessive disease names; for example, Crohn disease or Alzheimer disease, unless the physician uses the possessive form; for example, Crohn's disease or Alzheimer's disease.

24. PM military time is converted to civilian time by subtracting 1200. Dictated: The patient was seen at 1800 hours. Type: Patient was seen at 1800 hrs.

25. Use commas to separate groups of numbers with five digits or more; for example, 30,000.

26. Use commas to separate unrelated numerals; for example, "In January 1998, 4793 patients were seen in the emergency department."

27. Use Roman numerals for cancer stages, EKG limb leads, world wars, and Joe Doe III. Arabic numbers are now preferred for cranial nerves and diabetes types.

28. Noun: Return for *followup* in 2 weeks.

    Adjective: *Follow-up* EKGs were done.

NOTE: *followup* and *follow-up* are both acceptable spellings of the noun and adjectival forms; however, *followup* is now preferred.

29. Significant information should not be abbreviated. Uppercase all letters for DO NOT RESUSCITATE, NO MAYDAY, and NO CODE. Dictated: DNR. Type: DO NOT RESUSCITATE.

30. Lab data should always be abbreviated, even in the diagnosis.

31. Do not use acronyms in a diagnosis (with the exception of lab data) unless you cannot determine which meaning is correct. Dictated: COPD. Type: Chronic obstructive pulmonary disease.

32. Do not use a plus sign without a numeral. Dictated: Pulses ++ and equal. Type: Pulses +2 and equal.

33. Dictated: Alert and oriented times three. Type: Alert and oriented ×3.

34. A zero precedes a decimal fraction. Dictated: Xanax point 5 milligrams was prescribed. Type: Rx Xanax 0.5 mg.

35. A 30-character signature line should be placed 4 lines down from the end of the report/letter.

36. Do not type the dictator's initials following the signature line in reports or letters. Double-space and type the dictator's initials followed by a colon and the transcriptionist's initials in lowercased letters. EXAMPLE:

_____

Dooley R. Magnificent, MD

drm:ncg

cc: Elmoe J. Aloe, MD

37. Additional copies to physicians and others should be doubled-spaced after the transcriptionist's initials. Lowercased cc: for *courtesy copy* or xc: for *extra copy;* either is acceptable. See item 36.

SAMPLE MEDICAL REPORTS

HISTORY AND PHYSICAL

PATIENT: DOE, ALLISON A.   **LOCATION**: 567E
MR #: 8986453   **D**: 01/12/2003
ADMITTED: 01/12/2003   **T**: 01/12/2003
DISCHARGED: 00/00/0000   **SSN**: 555-55-5555
PHYSICIAN: JOHN Q. FIXIT, MD

HISTORY OF THE PRESENT ILLNESS: Patient is a very pleasant 61-year-old white female with a past medical history of interstitial cystitis and a mild anxiety disorder since the onset of the cystitis. She presented to the emergency department earlier today with a complaint of substernal chest pressure. She was given several sublingual nitroglycerin and did have improvement in her symptoms. An EKG revealed subtle ST-T wave changes in the anterior precordial leads. She was subsequently admitted for further evaluation. Repeat EKG revealed no significant change. Cardiac enzymes and other laboratory tests are still pending.

PAST MEDICAL/SURGICAL HISTORY: As above.

DRUG ALLERGIES: None known.

MEDICATIONS: Toprol XL 50 mg q.d., Xanax, Flexeril, and Elmiron for cystitis.

SOCIAL/FAMILY HISTORY: Noncontributory.

PHYSICAL EXAMINATION
VITAL SIGNS: Temperature 96, pulse 90, respirations 20, blood pressure 140/79.
GENERAL: Elderly-appearing white female in no acute distress. Alert and oriented ×3.
HEENT/NECK: Grossly unremarkable. No thyromegaly or carotid bruits.
HEART: Normal S1 and S2, soft S4 gallop, no S3. Occasional ectopic beat, 1 to 2/6 systolic murmur at the left sternal border.
LUNGS: Clear to auscultation and percussion. No rales, rhonchi, or wheezes.
ABDOMEN: Soft, nontender. No gross organomegaly or masses.
PELVIC/RECTAL: Deferred.
EXTREMITIES: No clubbing or cyanosis. There was mild bilateral pretibial edema. Pulses +2 bilaterally.

IMPRESSION: Chest pain and abnormal electrocardiogram with symptoms concerning for coronary artery disease.

PLAN: Admit to a monitored bed, rule out for myocardial infarction, and consider exercise stress testing versus cardiac catheterization pending cardiac enzymes.

_____

John Q. Fixit, MD

jqf:pjl

cc: Robert T. Feelgood, MD

HISTORY AND PHYSICAL

PATIENT: TIME, JUSTIN O.   **LOCATION**: 235W
MR #: 524789   **D**: 03/05/2003
ADMITTED: 03/05/2003   **T**: 03/05/2003
DISCHARGED: 00/00/0000   **SSN**: 555-55-5555
PHYSICIAN: I. M. ONCALL, MD

CHIEF COMPLAINT: Chest pain.

HISTORY OF PRESENT ILLNESS: Patient is a 65-year-old white man with coronary artery disease and prior PTCA stent to the left anterior descending branch. He has hyperlipidemia and parkinsonism. He does not have hypertension or diabetes mellitus. He had done well since his previous stent and, in fact, had a normal stress test 2 weeks ago as an outpatient. He reports retrosternal pressure-like discomfort radiating to neck, shoulder, and arm, with dyspnea and diaphoresis improved with nitroglycerin. He feels the discomfort today was more serious than that which he had at the time of his unstable angina prior to his stent placement. He has had no symptoms since that time. No dyspnea on exertion, nocturnal dyspnea, or orthopnea, but he has had lower extremity edema that is new. He denies tachyarrhythmias or syncope.

DRUG ALLERGIES: None known.

MEDICATIONS: Zocor 40 mg daily; Sinemet 25/100, 2 tablets t.i.d.; Ecotrin 325 mg daily; Seroquel 100 mg q.h.s.; clonazepam 0.25 mg b.i.d.; Prilosec 20 mg daily; amantadine 100 mg b.i.d.; Permax 1.05 mg t.i.d.; and nitroglycerin sublingually p.r.n. chest pain.

FAMILY HISTORY: Positive for coronary artery disease.

SOCIAL HISTORY: Patient does not use alcohol or tobacco. He is accompanied by his wife and daughter.

REVIEW OF SYSTEMS: HEAD/NECK: No transient ischemic attacks, stroke, head trauma, or seizure disorder, but he does have parkinsonism. GI: No melena, hematochezia, peptic ulcer disease, or gallbladder disease, but he has gastroesophageal reflux disease. RESPIRATORY: No fevers, chills, or productive cough. GU: No dysuria or hematuria. ENDOCRINE: Hyperlipidemia but no known diabetes mellitus or hypothyroidism. MUSCULOSKELETAL: He has no arthritis or degenerative joint disease. The remainder of the review of systems is negative except as stated above.

PHYSICAL EXAMINATION
VITAL SIGNS: Pulse 72, respirations 16, blood pressure 108/72, temperature 97.9.
GENERAL: Awake, alert, and oriented ×3, in no acute distress.
HEENT/NECK: Jugular venous pressure normal. Carotid pulses normal. No bruits. Thyroid not enlarged.
LUNGS: Clear bilaterally.
CARDIOVASCULAR: S1 and S2 normal. S4 gallop. No murmur, S3, or rub.
ABDOMEN: Bowel sounds normoactive. No tenderness or masses.
EXTREMITIES: No edema. Peripheral pulses intact bilaterally.
GENITORECTAL: Deferred.

DIAGNOSTIC STUDIES: EKG reveals sinus rhythm with premature atrial contractions and nondiagnostic ST-T wave abnormalities. CPK-MB 5.2.

HISTORY AND PHYSICAL

IMPRESSION
1. Unstable angina pectoris versus myocardial infarction secondary to #2.
2. Coronary artery disease.
3. Hyperlipidemia.
4. Parkinsonism.

RECOMMENDATIONS
1. Serial EKGs and cardiac enzymes.
2. Plavix, nitroglycerin, aspirin, and Lovenox.
3. Plan cardiac catheterization and possible angioplasty. The patient and his family understand the risks, including stroke, myocardial infarction, and possibility of bypass surgery, and wish to proceed.

_____

I. M. Oncall, MD

imo:oop

CONSULTATION

PATIENT: DOE, JOSEPH J.

MR #: 50089

ADMITTED: 01/02/2003

DISCHARGED: 00/00/0000

PHYSICIAN: LUCY FIXEMUP, MD

LOCATION: 895W

D: 01/02/2003

T: 01/02/2003

SSN: 555-55-5555

REASON FOR CONSULTATION: Management of atrial fibrillation.

HISTORY OF PRESENT ILLNESS: Patient is a 72-year-old white male who recently presented with an abdominal mass which was felt to be colon cancer. He was referred to Dr. Allwell for evaluation, and a walled-off diverticular abscess was found. A colostomy was deemed necessary, but hopefully, in about 2 to 3 months, he will be able to have the colostomy reversed.

PAST MEDICAL HISTORY: Significant for chronic atrial fibrillation with no other underlying coronary artery disease. He has had diverticulosis in the past and actually has done very well; he has no other chronic medical illnesses.

MEDICATIONS: Lanoxin 0.125 mg q.d., along with Coumadin 2.5 mg q.d. ×6 each week.

SOCIAL HISTORY: Divorced, retired. No smoking or alcohol use.

FAMILY HISTORY: Noncontributory.

REVIEW OF SYSTEMS: No shortness of breath, chest pain, or lightheadedness.

PHYSICAL EXAMINATION
GENERAL: Alert and oriented, in no acute distress.
VITAL SIGNS: BP 120/80, heart rate 83, irregularly irregular, afebrile.
SKIN: Warm and dry.
HEENT: Grossly normal.
LUNGS: Clear.
HEART: Irregularly irregular, without murmur, rub, or gallop.
ABDOMEN: Dressing is intact, with functioning colostomy.
GU/RECTAL: Deferred.
EXTREMITIES: Without edema.
NEUROLOGIC: Nonfocal.

DIAGNOSTIC STUDIES: EKG reveals chronic atrial fibrillation and incomplete right bundle branch block, which is unchanged from previous EKGs. Hemoglobin 13. PT 14.6. Yesterday, glucose was 241, calcium 7.3, magnesium 1.7, total bilirubin 1.4, GGTP 120. Urinalysis remarkable for a urobilinogen of 8.

ASSESSMENT/PLAN:

1. Chronic atrial fibrillation. Wean off Cardizem because his rate is now controlled and continue IV digoxin; switch to p.o. when able. Will put him on subcu Lovenox because he is stable postop; will resume his Coumadin orally at 5 mg q.d. and lower the dosage as soon as his PT is adjusted.

2. Increased glucose, probably related to intravenous fluids. Check fasting and 4 p.m. glucose to make sure it does not continue to be a problem.

Lucy Fixemup, MD

lf:jft

cc: Allen Sawbones, MD

CONSULTATION

PATIENT: DOE, MICHAEL H.

MR #: 561214

ADMITTED: 03/09/2003

DISCHARGED: 00/00/0000

PHYSICIAN: HUMU LYNN, MD

LOCATION: 987E

D: 03/10/2003

T: 03/11/2003

SSN: 555-55-5555

IDENTIFICATION DATA: This is a 51-year-old African American male currently admitted to Wecare Hospital. He is referred for psychiatric consultation. The information contained in this report is derived from a brief interview with this gentleman, as well as review of the record.

HISTORY OF PRESENT ILLNESS: This is a 51-year-old African American male who was admitted to WMC, transferred from a local jail facility after noted seizure activity. Initial documentation suggested the possibility of anoxic brain injury and encephalopathy, which by review of records, appeared to resolve over the early course of hospital stay. The ongoing problems have been the persistent report of auditory and visual hallucinations; history of pneumonia, which has been treated; diabetes mellitus; mild electrolyte abnormalities.

This patient reports that he has been seeing things such as snakes and other reptiles crawling about on his hospital room floor. He reports that this began to occur shortly after his admission to this facility and denies that hallucinations have occurred prior in his life. In addition, he reports that he will occasionally think the phone is ringing, only to pick it up and hear a dial tone. He states that occasionally he feels as though bugs are crawling on him. He denies previous history of mental illness or seeking out psychiatric services in the past. He did attend group meetings at a local church for alcohol abuse in the 1970s.

He does not appear to be frightened in any way by these hallucinations. They appear to occur randomly. At the time of interview, he does not appear to be actively hallucinating in any way.

CURRENT MEDICATIONS
1. Actos.
2. Flonase.
3. Insulin.
4. Toprol.
5. Risperdal.
6. Pepcid.

PAST MEDICAL/SURGICAL HISTORY: Known history of seizure disorder, currently taking Dilantin; diabetes; and previous cholecystectomy. He recently was diagnosed as having pneumonia, which has been treated.

MENTAL STATUS EXAMINATION: This gentleman is found to be alert. He is oriented in all spheres. There is no evidence of paranoid ideation. He is reporting intermittent episodes of visual hallucinations. He reports that most often these occur as a perception of snakes, other reptiles, and/or bugs crawling about the floor. These are not occurring presently. In addition, he reports auditory hallucinations in the form of hearing the phone ring only to answer it and find a dial tone. He is reporting tactile experiences as well. Judgment to hypotheticals appears marginally intact; judgment to recent real-life situations marginal. Concentration clearly diminished. Intelligence noted to be less than average. This gentleman appears to be quite concrete in his thinking. He is oriented to person and place only. He believes the month is June and the year is 1997. He also believes it is Saturday. There is no evidence of homicidal or suicidal thinking. Thought process generally goal directed.

CONSULTATION

INITIAL IMPRESSION

Axis I.	Psychosis, not otherwise specified.
Axis II.	Deferred.
Axis III.	Diabetes mellitus, seizure disorder, pneumonia status post treatment.
Axis IV.	Moderate.
Axis V.	At interview 45-50.

INITIAL RECOMMENDATION: This gentleman appears to be experiencing organic hallucinosis. To the best of his memory, onset followed admission to this facility. The record documents the possibility of seizure activity occurring at jail for some time. This gentleman denies drug use to me, although he does report alcohol consumption. I am certainly curious as to whether he experienced frank withdrawal while in jail and whether the seizure activity was part of that withdrawal syndrome. He apparently had some subsequent potential anoxic injury that appears, by review of record, to have slightly improved. This gentleman does not in any way appear to be frightened or alarmed by these hallucinatory experiences. I recommend consideration of a slight increase in his Risperdal. He appears to be tolerating this reasonably well. I would increase his dosage by 0.5 mg q.3-4d. up to about 2 mg p.o. total daily dose and hold at that dose. This gentleman is not likely to benefit from any inpatient psychiatric services at this time and continues to await further disposition and placement.

Humu Lynn, MD

hl:jjl

OPERATIVE REPORT

PATIENT: DOE, LARRY T.
MR #: 546845
DATE: 01/25/2003
PHYSICIAN: DEE CUBITUS, MD

LOCATION: 902E
D: 01/24/2003
T: 01/25/2003
SSN: 555-55-5555

PREOPERATIVE DIAGNOSIS(ES): Upper endoscopy with biopsies and brushings.

ATTENDING: Dr. Wincare

INDICATIONS FOR PROCEDURE: Patient with anemia and complaints of pain as well as heme-positive stools.

MEDICATIONS GIVEN: Versed 3 mg, Cetacaine spray.

DESCRIPTION OF THE PROCEDURE: After informed consent, discussing risks and benefits, including bleeding, infection, possible perforation, possibly missing a lesion, the patient was placed in the left lateral decubitus position. The oropharynx was sprayed with Cetacaine spray. A bite block was inserted without difficulty. The Olympus endoscope was passed through the bite block through the oropharynx into the esophagus. Within the esophagus, there was noted to be severe evidence of inflammation with what appeared to be candidal esophagitis in the mid-esophagus. Biopsies and brushings were obtained. In the distal esophagus was erythema and inflammation consistent with gastroesophageal reflux disease. The scope was advanced into the stomach, where vascular ectasia of the fundal portion of the stomach was noted. The scope was then advanced to the pylorus and first and second portions of the duodenum, which were essentially normal. The scope was then removed without difficulty. The patient tolerated the procedure well. There were no immediate complications. There were a total of 2 specimens taken, a brushing, and a biopsy from the esophagus.

IMPRESSION
1. Severe esophagitis, questionable Candida, although this appears likely.
2. Gastroesophageal reflux disease; biopsies, and brushings obtained.
3. Vascular ectasia in the fundus, which is probably the cause of the patient's bleeding; however, colonoscopy is still warranted given his heme-positive stools.

PLAN
1. Proton pump inhibitor b.i.d.
2. Check biopsies.
3. Colonoscopy.

On behalf of my colleagues, I would like to thank Dr. Wincare for allowing me to participate in this patient's care.

_____

Dee Cubitus, MD

dc:mit

DISCHARGE SUMMARY

PATIENT: DOE, ARNOLD M.
MR #: 98385
ADMITTED: 01/05/2003
DISCHARGED: 01/09/2003
PHYSICIAN: JACK T. OUCH, MD

LOCATION: DISCHARGED
D: 01/09/2003
T: 01/10/2003
SSN: 555-55-5555

DICTATED BY: Angela Feelbetter, ACNP-CS

DISCHARGE DIAGNOSES
1. Chronic obstructive pulmonary disease exacerbation.
2. Coronary artery disease.
3. Dyslipidemia.
4. Epigastric pain.
5. Alcohol abuse.

DISCHARGE MEDICATIONS
1. Lescol 40 mg every day.
2. Combivent metered dose inhaler, 2 puffs b.i.d.
3. Norvasc 5 mg every day.
4. Zantac 300 mg q.h.s.
5. Lasix 20 mg every day.
6. Toprol XL 50 mg every day.
7. Atrovent inhaler 2 puffs t.i.d. p.r.n.
8. Serax 15 mg b.i.d.

HISTORY: Patient is a 76-year-old Caucasian male who presented to the emergency department on the day of admission with an acute onset of dyspnea. At approximately 5:00 a.m. the morning of admission, he experienced difficulty breathing and had to crawl upstairs to summon help from his wife. He denied chest pain but admitted that 4 days prior to admission, he had a 2-day history of diarrhea that has since resolved. He has had epigastric pain as well. He was recently seen by me in the office within the past month with complaints of abdominal pain. Laboratory findings at that time were unremarkable, and a CT of the abdomen did not reveal any acute process. The patient has a longstanding history of alcohol abuse, primarily drinking scotch, and it was uncertain how much alcohol he had been consuming before his admission. While being examined in the emergency department, he had an episode of supraventricular tachycardia, at which time he related he felt dizzy. This was similar to how he felt on the morning of admission. He also was noted to have sinus tachycardia persistently with episodes of bigeminy as well. Please refer to the H & P for further information.

LABORATORY DATA: On the date of admission, ABG on 3 liter nasal cannula revealed pH 7.54, Pco_2 25.9, Po_2 83.6, bicarbonate 22.1, O_2 saturation 97.2%. HGB 15.2, HCT 45.1, WBCs 5.5, platelets 164,000. Differential within normal limits with the exception of 5% eosinophils. Sodium 140, potassium 3.6, chloride 102, CO_2 of 23, BUN 9, creatinine 1.1, glucose 102, magnesium 1.8. AMI profile negative ×3 for myocardial injury. Theophylline level 9.0 on admission. Urinalysis within normal limits. Chest x-ray revealed COPD but no acute cardiopulmonary disease evident. EKG on admission revealed normal sinus rhythm with borderline 1st degree AV block, left-axis deviation, anterior fascicular block, and possible old anterior infarct. Echocardiogram on admission was a technically poor study. No definite anterior infarct. No definite valvular abnormalities were noted.

DISCHARGE SUMMARY

HOSPITAL COURSE: Patient was admitted to the Progressive Care Unit and a myocardial infarction was in fact ruled out. A Holter monitor was placed, and report is pending at time of dictation. CIWA protocol was instituted given his history of ETOH abuse; however, he did not experience frank DTs. He did have problems with tremulousness, which did abate to some extent. It was uncertain as to whether this resolved secondary to initiation of Serax or discontinuation of his Uniphyl. He remained normal sinus rhythm with intermittent 1st degree AV block and no other dysrhythmias during his stay on the PCU. His pulmonary status improved with no further problems of dyspnea and no chest pain. He persisted with some epigastric burning throughout the course of his stay, but this was better than on admission. By January 5, 2003, he was ambulating without difficulty and had improved to baseline.

DISPOSITION: Discharged to home. Patient is alert and oriented and considered capable of handling his own affairs. He will follow up with me in the office in 2 weeks. No activity restrictions. Patient is instructed to follow a low cholesterol diet as previously.

PROCEDURES: None.

CONSULTATIONS: None.

_____

Jack T. Ouch, MD

Dictated by Angela Feelbetter

jto:pjl

cc: Sam S. Suture, MD

TRANSFER SUMMARY

PATIENT: DOE, JULIANNA M.   **LOCATION**: DISCHARGED
MR #: 98385   **D**: 02/12/2003
ADMITTED: 02/07/2003   **T**: 02/12/2003
DISCHARGED: 02/12/2003   **SSN**: 555-55-5555
PHYSICIAN: BILLY RUBIN, MD

HISTORY OF PRESENT ILLNESS: This is a 75-year-old Caucasian female with ulcerative colitis who presented to the emergency department with nausea, vomiting, and diarrhea. These symptoms had been present for 3 days. She presented to the emergency department, was found to be hypokalemic, and was admitted for further treatment with IV fluids and potassium replacement. She does have a history of atherosclerotic heart disease with poor left ventricular function and history of congestive heart failure.

PHYSICAL EXAMINATION: Please see H & P.

LABORATORY DATA: HGB 13.3, HCT 39.4, and WBCs 6100. Follow-up hemoglobin was in the range of 12.3 to 12.6. CMET was normal except for a random glucose of 124, potassium 2.8, and albumin 3.2. Follow-up potassium normalized to 4.1-4.4. Lanoxin level was 0.6. Stool for Clostridium difficile was negative. Stool for Giardia and Cryptosporidium was negative. Stool for blood was positive. Stool culture showed normal fecal flora with no Salmonella-Shigella or Campylobacter. Chest x-ray showed cardiomegaly with no congestive heart failure. Abdominal x-rays showed increased gaseous distention in the colon. Follow-up abdominal x-rays after rectal tube was placed did show improvement in gaseous distention. EKG revealed sinus rhythm with frequent PVCs, left-axis deviation, and intraventricular conduction delay.

HOSPITAL COURSE: Patient was initially admitted to the PCU. She was started on IV fluids and given supplemental potassium. She was placed on Solu-Medrol IV rather than her p.o. prednisone. She was restarted on Asacol. Her nausea, vomiting, and distended abdomen had resolved. She had improvement in her diarrhea, but her diarrhea never really went away during the hospitalization. She had poor p.o. intake during the hospitalization, stating that she was just not hungry and did not want to eat. She did not want a feeding tube. She maintained her hydration level without developing evidence of dehydration. However, she is at risk for dehydration with her need for Lasix to keep her out of congestive heart failure. She has not been asking for her Imodium very often, and I think a trial of routine Imodium would be the next step to see if it will help check her diarrhea to some degree. She has reached maximum hospital benefit, considering that she does not want any further aggressive treatment such as a feeding tube. The patient's sister is reluctant to place her in an extended care facility but understands that there is not really anything else that we can do here at the hospital.

FINAL DIAGNOSES
1. Ulcerative colitis.
2. Anorexia with poor intake.
3. Hypokalemia, resolved.
4. Atherosclerotic heart disease with poor left ventricular function and history of congestive heart failure.
5. Premature ventricular contractions.
6. Osteoporosis.
7. History of seizures.

DISPOSITION: Transferred to the nursing home facility on Asacol 400 mg t.i.d.; two aspirin 81 mg q.a.m.; Lanoxin 0.25 mg q.a.m.; Aricept 5 mg q.a.m.; Pepcid 20 mg q.a.m.; Prozac 20 mg q.a.m.; nitroglycerin patch to the skin q.a.m. and removed at 10 p.m.; K-Dur 20 mEq b.i.d.; prednisone 30 mg q.a.m.; and

TRANSFER SUMMARY

Imodium 2 mg b.i.d. She also has Phenergan 12.5 mg q.4h. p.r.n. nausea. Her prednisone should be tapered to 20 mg daily in 1 week and 10 mg daily after another week. Imodium should be held if she develops constipation. If she continues to have poor p.o. intake and appears to be getting dehydrated, her Lasix should be held.

PROGNOSIS: Poor. Patient is not eating well and does not want a feeding tube.

_____

Billy Rubin, MD

br:ccg

TRANSFER SUMMARY

PATIENT: BENINPAIN, TINA J.   **LOCATION**: 235W
MR #: 1234568   **D**: 02/05/2002
ADMITTED: 02/02/2002   **T**: 02/05/2002
DISCHARGED: 00/00/0000   **SSN**: 555-55-5555
PHYSICIAN: ART E. OGRAPHY, MD

DICTATED BY: Nancy Nitroglycerin, ACNP-CS

FINAL DIAGNOSES

1. Myocardial infarction.
2. Coronary artery disease.
   a) History of previous coronary artery bypass grafting in 1986 with left internal mammary of the LAD and saphenous vein graft to the obtuse marginal.
   b) Status post left heart catheterization with graft arteriography, March 5, 2003, with the results as follows:
      1) Left internal mammary artery of the LAD and saphenous vein graft to obtuse marginal patent.
      2) There is 60 to 70% stenosis in the RCA, proximal.
      3) Left circumflex totally occluded.
      4) LAD with 85% stenosis in the distal vessel involving the 3rd diagonal.
      5) Ejection fraction 50%.
   c) Patient transferred to Heartcare Hospital to undergo PCI of the RCA.
3. Hypertension.
4. History of vasovagal syncope. Negative EP study, June 2001.
5. History of gastrointestinal bleeding, June 25, 2001, with EGD demonstrating hiatal hernia with esophageal erosions and ulcerations and mild antral gastritis.
6. History of repair of right femoral pseudoaneurysm in 1997.
7. Chronic right lower extremity edema.
8. Remote history of deep vein thrombosis.
9. Right bundle branch block.
10. History of cholecystectomy and hiatal hernia with left rib resection.

TRANSFER MEDICATIONS

1. Mucomyst 600 mg b.i.d.
2. Enteric-coated aspirin 325 mg daily.
3. Lovenox 79 mg b.i.d.
4. Lopressor 25 mg b.i.d.
5. Protonix 40 mg b.i.d.
6. Demadex 20 mg every other day alternating with 10 mg.
7. Half normal saline 50 cc/hr.
8. Integrilin 2 mcg/kg/min.
9. Nitroglycerin infusion.

PROCEDURES: Left heart catheterization with graft arteriography, March 5, 2002.

TRANSFER SUMMARY

CONSULTATIONS: None.

LABORATORY DATA: Chemistries, March 7, 2002, demonstrate sodium 137, potassium 3.8, chloride 103, CO_2 of 24, BUN 22, creatinine 1.8, glucose 96. CBC on March 4, 2002, demonstrates WBCs 9.9, HGB 13.8, HCT 41.6, platelets 315,000. Cardiac enzymes demonstrated a peak troponin 6.6. CK-MB peaked at 11.1. CT scan of the head was unremarkable. Chest x-ray demonstrated ectasia of the aortic arch. The heart was at the upper limits of normal. Lungs were clear. CT of the chest was negative for pulmonary embolus and aortic dissection. EKG was markedly abnormal, demonstrating a sinus rhythm with right bundle branch block and diffuse T wave inversion.

HOSPITAL COURSE: This patient is a 77-year-old gentleman with known coronary artery disease admitted to the Wecare Medical Center on March 4, 2002, with chest pain with some atypical features for angina. His initial cardiac enzymes were mildly elevated. He was admitted for observation. CT scan of the chest was negative for pulmonary embolus and aortic dissection. He underwent repeat cardiac catheterization on March 5, 2002, with results as noted above. We initially elected for medical therapy, but the patient had recurrent chest pain and he is transferred now to Heartcare Hospital on March 7, 2002, to undergo PCI of the right coronary artery under Dr. Angieo's care.

DISPOSITION: This patient is transferred to the Heartcare Hospital to undergo PTCA/stent of the right coronary artery. The risks and benefits of the procedure have been discussed with the patient and his daughter, and they are in agreement to proceed. Transfer medications are as above. Diet is low fat, low cholesterol, low sodium.

Art E. Ography, MD

aeo:ccg

cc: Kineso Therapee, MD

RADIOLOGY REPORT

PATIENT: TREATME, AUSTIN   **LOCATION**: 756W
MR #: 32568   **D**: 02/04/2003
DATE: 02/04/2003   **T**: 02/04/2003
PHYSICIAN: LUTHER T. X-RAY, MD   **SSN**: 555-55-5555

CLINICAL DATA: Pain in the left knee and hip.

LEFT FEMUR: Two views of the left femur were obtained. There is an acute left-sided intertrochanteric femoral neck fracture. There is varus angulation at the fracture site. The femoral head remains located within the acetabulum. The bones are mildly osteopenic.

IMPRESSION: Acute left intertrochanteric femoral neck fracture with varus angulation at the fracture site.

AP CHEST: Single AP view of the chest was obtained without prior studies for comparison. The patient is rotated to the right. The lungs are hyperinflated with flattening of the hemidiaphragms. The heart size is within normal limits. The lungs are clear of focal infiltrates, effusions, and pneumothoraces.

IMPRESSION: Chronic changes of chronic obstructive pulmonary disease and atherosclerosis. Otherwise, no evidence of acute pulmonary disease.

_____

Luther T. X-ray, MD

ltx:jjj

RADIOLOGY REPORT

PATIENT: BENAHURT, CYNTHIA   **LOCATION**: 456W
MR #: 85945   **D**: 02/04/2003
DATE: 02/04/2003   **T**: 02/04/2003
PHYSICIAN: RAY D. OLOGY, MD   **SSN**: 555-55-5555

CLINICAL DATA: Renal dysfunction.

RENAL ULTRASOUND: Portable study was carried out in the ICU and is quite limited as a result. However, both kidneys were demonstrated. The lower pole of the left kidney appears to contain a 2.7 cm mass. This is either anechoic or hypoechoic and could represent either a cyst or a solid mass with low-level echoes. The right kidney appears unremarkable, measuring 10.1 cm in sagittal dimension. There was no evidence of hydronephrosis. No shadowing stones were demonstrated.

IMPRESSION: The study was limited due to portable technique as described. There was a mass effect at the lower pole of the left kidney. I suggest reevaluating this with ultrasound in the Radiology Department when the patient's condition permits; if that does not clarify the character of this structure, then multi-phase CT will be needed.

_____

Ray D. Ology, MD

rdo:mmm

PATHOLOGY REPORT

PATIENT: DOREME, DELORIS   **LOCATION**: 675W
MR #: 21565   **D**: 01/14/2003
DATE: 01/14/2003   **T**: 01/15/2003
PHYSICIAN: STAN Q. SURGERY, MD   **SSN**: 555-55-5555

SPECIMEN: Left breast, targeted needle biopsy.

CLINICAL INFORMATION: Left lower outer quadrant mammographic mass density lesion, estimated size 6.4 × 6.0 mm; U/S-guided biopsy of 2 specimens. Clinical working diagnosis is invasive cancer, low-grade invasive ductal.

*MACROSCOPIC DESCRIPTION: By standard procedure, each biopsy core is immediately formalin-spritzed from the needle into 10% NBF. The biopsies are received from the lab, being approximately 2 needle biopsies or mammotome cores, and possibly some additional small fragments, which are gray-white to yellow. Altogether, the biopsy aggregate measures approximately 1.0 × 0.4 × 0.2 cm. It is placed into a screen cassette, into the magnetic stirrer with 10% NBF and totally processed in 1 block. HM/xyz January 3, 2000.

MICROSCOPIC DESCRIPTION: Sections show invasive ductal carcinoma with cords, nests, and tubules infiltrating in a sclerotic stroma (2 points for tubule formation). Tumor cells show relatively uniform small nuclei (1.5 RBC size) without prominent nucleoli and diffuse chromatin pattern (nuclear grade I). Mitosis is not readily detected (1 point for mitotic rate). This is a total of 4 points, Elston tumor grade I, well differentiated. There is no tumor necrosis in the invasive component. Focal cribriform DCIS is identified with rare micro-focal necrosis. No peritumoral vascular/lymphatic invasion is seen. Ancillary tests are reserved for resection section.

DIAGNOSTIC OPINION: Left breast, needle core biopsy: invasive ductal carcinoma, well differentiated (Elston tumor grade I). (174.9)

_____

Stan Q. Surgery, MD

sqs:ofh

---

*MACROSCOPIC DESCRIPTION formerly GROSS DESCRIPTION.

CAROTID ULTRASOUND REPORT

PATIENT: DOE, ADEAR A.   **LOCATION**: OUTPATIENT
MR #: 98385   **D**: 02/17/2003
DATE: 02/17/2003   **T**: 02/18/2003
PHYSICIAN: SUE DOCYST, MD   **SSN**: 555-55-5555

CLINICAL INFORMATION: This is a 78-year-old female who had a previous right carotid endarterectomy in 1995. The patient has no current symptoms but is having a repeat study for follow-up.

FINDINGS: There is evidence of the previous graft on the right side, and there is no evidence of any luminal obstruction on the right. There is mild atherosclerotic plaquing at the origins of both left ICA and left ECA and moderate atherosclerosis in the mid left ICA, but none of these plaques significantly obstruct the lumen. The peak systolic and end diastolic velocities are in an acceptable range. There is fairly significant tortuosity of the vessel, especially on the left side. Antegrade flow is noted in the right vertebral. No flow can be documented in the left vertebral.

FINAL IMPRESSION

1. Previous right carotid endarterectomy with patch-graft.
2. Atherosclerotic plaquing to a moderate degree in the left mid internal carotid artery, but no intraluminal stenosis.
3. No hemodynamically significant stenosis by spectral or velocity criteria.
4. Antegrade flow in the right vertebral and no flow detected in the left vertebral.
5. Since the previous study of August 1, 2002, the left vertebral artery shows no flow, but otherwise the study is unchanged.

_____

Sue Docyst, MD

sd:aah

EMERGENCY DEPARTMENT NOTE

PATIENT: DALL, HAL

MR #: 98385

ADMITTED: 02/24/2003

DISCHARGED: 02/24/2003

PHYSICIAN: U.R. WELL, MD

LOCATION: ER3

D: 02/24/2003

T: 02/24/2003

SSN: 555-55-5555

CHIEF COMPLAINT: Tongue swelling.

HISTORY OF PRESENT ILLNESS: Patient is a 43-year-old male who states he has had a history of anxiety, depression, and mood swings. He indicates he was seen by his primary care physician 2 days ago and given Haldol. He states he did not take any Haldol yesterday, but this morning when he woke up he felt like his tongue was thick and he had difficulty opening his mouth. Throughout the evening he felt very "jittery" and was unable to sleep. Denies any headache, fevers, chest pain, back pain, abdominal pain, or other extremity pain.

REVIEW OF SYSTEMS: Constitutional, ENT, ophthalmologic, cardiac, respiratory, GI, GU, hematologic, oncologic, neurologic, psychiatric, musculoskeletal, integument, and endocrine all reviewed and negative except for that mentioned above.

PAST MEDICAL/SURGICAL HISTORY: Noncontributory.

DRUG ALLERGIES: PENICILLIN.

CURRENT MEDICATIONS: Xanax and just started on Paxil.

PHYSICAL EXAMINATION: GENERAL: Well-developed, well-nourished male. VITAL SIGNS: Temperature 97, pulse 90, respiratory rate 18, blood pressure 129/94, O_2 saturation 98%. HEENT: PERRLA. EOMI. TMs negative. Nares clear. Oropharynx, the patient is holding his mouth in open position with his tongue swollen; however, there is no evidence of lingual, buccal, or uvular swelling and no stridor. LUNGS: Clear. CARDIAC: Regular rate and rhythm. Normal S1 and S2. No gallops, rubs, or murmurs appreciated. ABDOMEN: Positive bowel sounds, soft and nontender. No organomegaly. No masses. SKIN: No rash, petechiae, or purpura. NEUROLOGIC: Cranial nerves 2-12 are intact. Motor 5/5 in all muscle groups.

MEDICAL DECISION MAKING: The patient appears to have dystonic reaction. I do not believe this is angioedema. He has no evidence of soft tissue, lingual, or pharyngeal swelling. No evidence of compromised airway.

ED COURSE: Patient was given Benadryl 50 mg IV and Cogentin 2 mg p.o. with complete resolution of his symptoms. I have discussed with the patient that it is extremely important not to take the Haldol. Likewise, I have suggested that he stop Paxil. Patient verbalized understanding. I have placed him on Cogentin for the next couple of days until Haldol clears from his system.

CLINICAL IMPRESSION: Dystonic reaction.

DISPOSITION: Discharged on Rx Cogentin 2 mg 1 p.o. q.12h. (#5). Return with more episodes of tongue swelling. No medications except Xanax. Follow up with physician on Monday. Take Cogentin until completed.

U. R. Well, MD

urw:plh

SOAP NOTE

PATIENT: BENACOUFIN, LORI A.   **D**: 02/14/2003
MR #: 546845   **T**: 02/15/2003
DATE: 02/14/2003   **SSN**: 555-55-5555
PHYSICIAN: MACK ROBIOTIC, MD

S: The patient is a 45-year-old white female complaining of a 1-week history of sore throat, swelling on the left side of the neck, and some aches. She has not noticed any fever but has been nauseated. ROS: As above, otherwise negative for congestion, cough, chest pain. CURRENT MEDS: None. ALLERGIES: None known. PMH/PSH: Noncontributory.

O: VITAL SIGNS: Temp 98.1, pulse 88/regular, respirations 16/unlabored, blood pressure 90/68. HEENT: Nasal septal deviation to the right. Ears with some fluid bilaterally. Throat shows erythema, no exudate. NECK: Bilateral anterior cervical lymphadenopathy with node masses measuring up to 2.5 cm in diameter. LUNGS: Clear to A & P. LAB DATA: Positive rapid strep screen. TX: Bicillin LA 1.2 million units IM and Phenergan IM for nausea.

A: Strep pharyngitis.

P: Decongestant of choice ×10 days. Rx Phenergan (#12, no refill). Follow up if symptoms do not improve or become worse.

_____
Mack Robiotic, MD

mr:ppo

SOAP NOTE (ADHESIVE)

EDEMA, ANGIE   12345   TURE/aaa   02/10/2003

S: Patient complains of nonproductive cough, clear rhinorrhea, and some head congestion. No sore throat. Feeling tired and slightly nauseated. She has been taking OTC Sudafed with little relief. She is having sneezing fits in the morning. No fever. MEDS: Sudafed and Cozaar h.s. PMH: Allergies and hypertension with blood pressures running between the 140s to 160s systolic.

O: GENERAL: No distress. VITAL SIGNS: Temperature 98.3, pulse 80/regular, respirations 18/unlabored, blood pressure 160/100. HEENT: TMs slightly retracted. Nasal mucosa mildly edematous. Clear rhinorrhea. Pharynx reveals some cobblestoning. No tonsillar enlargement. No exudate. No sinus tenderness noted. NECK: Supple, no adenopathy. HEART: Regular rate and rhythm without murmur. LUNGS: Clear.

A: 1. Viral upper respiratory infection with underlying allergies.
    2. Hypertension.

P: Switch Cozaar to Hyzaar 50/12.5 (samples given 1 month). Zyrtec 10 mg. p.o. daily (#10 samples and #30, refill ×3). Aquatab DM 1 p.o. b.i.d. p.r.n. cough (#20 no refill). Work excuse given. Follow up in 1 month for BP check.

CARE, JANE   45658   TURE/aaa   02/10/2003

S: Patient complains of substernal chest pain and describes it as an "ache" that comes and goes ×1 month. Pain lasts for a few seconds then spontaneously goes away. There is no association of the pain with eating, activity, stress level, positioning. Motrin tends to ease the pain, but the pain returns. She states it is somewhat sore to touch in the anterior and posterior chest. She has a history of heart palpitations, but they are very insignificant at this time. Patient is a smoker but has greatly decreased the number of cigarettes smoked per day. She had an upper respiratory infection approximately 1 month ago and had a good deal of coughing spells. She has noticed an increase in her back and flank pain with slouching at her desk job. EKG in February showed borderline bundle branch block and Holter monitor showed some SVT. MEDS: Celexa. No family history of early onset of cardiac disease.

O: GENERAL: No distress. Conversation and affect appropriate. Afebrile. HEART: Grade 2/6 systolic murmur located in the tricuspid area. LUNGS: Clear. MUSCULOSKELETAL: No tenderness on palpation along the vertebral nor on the trapezius bilaterally. No pain or tenderness on palpation of the anterior chest wall. LAB: Chest x-ray within normal limits. H & H, WBCs, and lymphocytes within normal limits. EKG revealed normal sinus rhythm, 80s to 90s with no acute abnormality.

A: Atypical chest pain, probably musculoskeletal in origin.

P: Anaprox 550 mg. p.o. b.i.d. p.r.n. pain (#60 no refill). Patient to contact me this week if symptoms are not relieved by the antiinflammatory, in which case we will set her up for a stress echo. If symptoms worsen despite treatment with antiinflammatory, she is to call the office immediately or go to the ER.

DOE, CARRIE   45658   TURE/aaa   02/10/2003

S: Patient complains of headaches and refill on medication. She has had an increase of headaches this week due to stress involving her daughter. This stress has been going on for approximately a year. States she took Imitrex and states she "felt funny in the head." Patient states she believes she has high cholesterol and heard on the TV people with high cholesterol should not take Imitrex. LDL was 115, HDL 67 2/01. She has a history of glaucoma, but this was normal at her last ophthalmology visit and she is not taking any current meds. She is due back for ophthalmology visit in April. Patient has tried antidepressants in the past for her mood and states she is "allergic to them" because they make her feel "disconnected." She also wishes to have LFTs done because she has been placed on Lamisil for onychomycosis. She had been on this for approximately 1 month but ran out of her prescription about 2 weeks ago and has not gotten it refilled. She also needs refills on Synthroid and Premarin because she has had a MMG in the past year, which was normal per her report. Regarding headaches, they are mainly temporal in origin, usually one-sided, and can turn into a migraine at some point. Imitrex gives some relief. She has been able to take 2 Fioricet a day for the past month. She has not sought the care of a neurologist for these headaches.

O: GENERAL: No acute distress. Conversation appropriate, somewhat argumentative, affect is flat. VITAL SIGNS: Temperature afebrile, blood pressure 130/70. HEENT: Nasal mucosal benign. Funduscopic benign. PERRLA. No temporal tenderness. NECK: Carotids 2+ equal bilaterally. No adenopathy or thyromegaly. CARDIAC: Regular rate and rhythm. LUNGS: Clear bilaterally. BACK: Some tenderness along the trapezius and lumbar areas. LAB DATA: Blood work drawn and pending, including a CBC to rule out borderline anemia. Urinalysis clear.

A: Tension headache, borderline anemia, menopause, hypothyroidism, and questionable drug dependency.

P: I spoke with the patient at length about continuing to take Fioricet and informed her that I do not agree with continuing to refill this medication as many times as we have in the past. I explained that we will give her a small amount today and she will be given a referral to either a neurologist or pain clinic. I suspect somewhat of a drug dependence in this patient. Encouraged patient to refill her Lamisil. Rx Synthroid 0.125 mg 1 p.o. every day (#90, no refill). Rx Premarin 0.9 mg 1 p.o. every day (#90, no refill). She does not need any Imitrex. Consider addition of antidepressant medication if stress headaches continue to increase. She is to follow up with Dr. Feelgood.

ADDENDUM: At the end of the visit, the patient requested a B-6 shot, which she received before leaving the office.

USA FAMILY PRACTICE
123 Main St.
Anywhere, IL 62294
(618) 555-5555

Alan Togenesis, MD	**Polly Pectomy, MD**
Al Veoli, CFNP	**Sue Ture, FNP-CS**
Billy Rubin, MD	**Angie Ography, PA**
Dee Cubitus, MD	**Bob Feelgood, MD**

February 27, 2003

John Busy, MD
1000 Candycane Lane
Sugarhill, NJ 22222

RE: Rita Doe
CHART #:   11111

Dear Dr. Busy:

Enclosed please find copies of Ms. Rita Doe's medical records. I saw Ms. Doe on September 10, 2001, and diagnosed her with acute anxiety in conjunction with situational depression, which may have an endogenous component. I believe that in addition to medical and psychological therapy, medical leave from work would be appropriate; work seems to be her main stressor. If possible, I would appreciate you seeing this patient within the next 3 to 4 weeks.

Thank you for your consideration of this matter. If I may be of further assistance, please do not hesitate to contact me.

With kindness personal regards, I am,

Sincerely yours,

Alan Togenesis, MD

at:wxy

enc

LETTERHEAD
555 Allie Lane
Superville, USA 88888
(888) 555-4329

February 2, 2003

To Whom It May Concern:

RE: Jonathan Doe

Mr. Doe is a 57-year-old African American male who was admitted to the hospital on January 2, 2003, and left the hospital on January 6, 2003. He had a diagnosis of acute stroke and has been followed in the office ever since. The last time he was in the office to see me was January 30, 2003.

The patient has multiple medical problems, including stroke, hypertension with ventricular systolic dysfunction with an ejection fraction of 35-40%, diabetes mellitus type 2, hypercholesterolemia, and proteinuria. Patient is able to carry light duty at his job.

If you have any questions, please contact my office at (999) 555-1234.

Sincerely,

Phil O. Progenitive, MD

pop:ae

TABLE **1-1** Microsoft Word Keyboard Shortcuts*

MENU	SHORTCUT
EDIT MENU	
Select	Hold Shift while moving cursor with arrow keys
Select All	Control a
Copy	Control c
Cut	Control x
Paste	Control v
Undo	Control z
Find	Control f
Display Nonprinting Info	Control *
VIEW MENU	
Normal view	Alt Ctrl n
Print Layout view	Alt Ctrl p or Ctrl F2
FORMAT MENU	
Bold	Ctrl b
Italic	Ctrl i
Underline	Ctrl u
Double underline	Ctrl Shift d
Word underline	Ctrl Shift w
Center align	Ctrl e
Justify	Ctrl j
Left align	Ctrl l
Hanging indent	Ctrl r
Unhang indent	Ctrl Shift t
FORCING THE ISSUE	
Nonbreaking hyphen	Ctrl Shift Hyphen
Nonbreaking space	Ctrl Shift Space
Page break	Ctrl Enter

*Note that Macintosh computers have different shortcut commands.

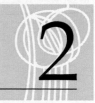

Medical Terminology

PREFIXES AND SUFFIXES

PREFIX OR SUFFIX	MEANING
a-	without
ab-	away from
-ac, -al	pertaining or relating to
ad-	toward, in the direction of
-algia	pain
ante-	before, toward
anti-	against
-ary	pertaining to
bi-	two
-cele	tumor, cyst, hernia
-centesis	surgical procedure, removal of fluid
-desis	binding together
-dynia	pain
dys-	difficult, painful
-ectomy	surgical removal
-ectasis	stretching, enlargement
-emia	blood condition
-esthesia	feeling, sensation
-gram	result of film or record
-graphy	process of recording
hemi-	half
homo-	same
hyper-	excessive, over, high
hypo-	low, decreased
intra-	within

-itis	inflammation
-lysis	destruction, to separate
-malacia	abnormal softening
-megaly	large, great
nulli-	none
-ologist	specialist
-ology	study of
-oma	tumor, mass
-osis	disease, abnormal condition
-otomy	incision, cutting
-pathy	disease
peri-	around
-pexy	surgical fixation
-plasty	surgical repair
-plegia	paralysis
-pnea	breathing
primi-	first
poly-	many
post-	after
pre-	before
-ptosis	drooping
-rrhage	bursting forth
-rrhaphy	to suture
-rrhea	discharge, flow
-rrhexis	rupture
-sclerosis	abnormal hardening
-scopy	visual examination
-stenosis	narrowing
sub-	below
super-, supra-	above, excessive
trans-	across, through
-tripsy	to crush
-uria	urine, urination

COMBINING FORMS

COMBINING FORM	MEANING
aden/o	gland
adip/o	fat
angi/o	vessel
arteri/o	artery
arthr/o	joint
blephar/o	eyelid
cardi/o	heart
cephal/o	head
cervic/o	neck
chol/e	gall
chondr/o	cartilage
cost/o	rib
crani/o	skull
cyst/o	bladder, sac
cyt/o	cell
dermat/o	skin
encephal/o	brain
gastr/o	stomach
hemat/o	blood
hepat/o	liver
hyster/o, uter/o	uterus
leuk/o	white
lip/o	fat
lith/o	stone
metr/o	uterine tissue
my/o	muscle
myel/o	bone marrow, spinal cord
nephr/o, ren/o	kidney
neur/o	nerve
oophor/o	ovary

ophthalm/o	eye
oste/o	bone
pharyng/o	pharynx, throat
pneumon/o, pulmon/o	lungs
py/o	pus
pyel/o	pelvis of kidney
rhin/o, nas/o	nasal tissue, nose
salping/o	fallopian tubes
splen/o	spleen
thorac/o	thorax, chest
thromb/o	clot
ureter/o	ureter

COMMONLY USED MEDICAL TERMS

TERM	MEANING
ache	persistent pain
acute	brief course; not chronic
afebrile	without fever
allergy	symptoms caused by sensitivity to a substance
ambulate	walk about
anomaly	deviation from the normal standard
aseptic	clean
atraumatic	without trauma
atrophy	wasting
benign	not malignant
bimanual	using both hands
cachectic	body wasting, weight loss, due to disease or emotional state
calcification	calcium deposit
catheter	tubular instrument used for passage of fluid or air
chronic	long term
congenital	existing at birth
constriction	tightening, narrowing
contaminate	unclean
contraindicated	inadvisable
crisis	sudden change
debris	foreign material that does not belong in an area

dehydration	reduction of body water content
demyelinization	loss of myelin
diaphoresis	perspiration
dilate	to enlarge
disease	dysfunction of body system, organs, illness
disposition	treatment/management
dyspnea	breathing difficulty
elicit	reveal
etiology	cause of disease
febrile	increased body temperature
fingerbreadth	width of a finger
hypertrophy	organ enlargement
immobile	no movement
infection	area invasion by microorganisms
inflamed	pain, warmth, swelling, or redness (tissue reaction)
malignant	destroy, harm, or may cause death
metastasis	spreading of disease to other body parts
mobile	movement
morbid	state of disease
necrosis	death of tissue
obese	excessive fatty tissue
occluded	closed
organomegaly	enlargement of organs
postural	pertaining to position
prognosis	probable outcome
prophylaxis	prevent spread of disease
prosthesis	artificial substitute for missing body part
provisional	temporary
purulent	pus containing substance
quadrant	quarter section
radiate	to spread
regimen	scheduled plan
retention	to keep/retain
sensitivity	to respond
septic	unclean
specimen	sample
stenosis	narrowing

sterile	germ free
stricture	narrowing of hollow structure
suture	to stitch with thread-like material
symptom	sign
syndrome	group of signs or symptoms
therapy	treatment
tract	pathway
trauma	injury
ulcer	lesion caused by superficial loss of tissue, inflammation usually occurs

Physical Examination Terms

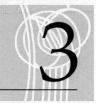

GENERAL TERMS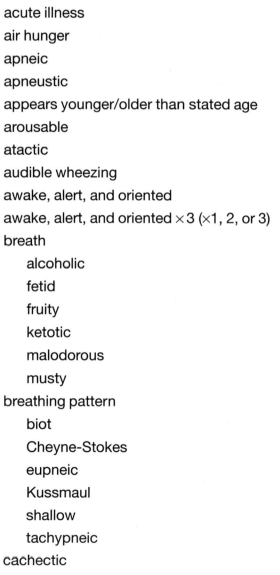

acute illness

air hunger

apneic

apneustic

appears younger/older than stated age

arousable

atactic

audible wheezing

awake, alert, and oriented

awake, alert, and oriented × 3 (×1, 2, or 3)

breath

    alcoholic

    fetid

    fruity

    ketotic

    malodorous

    musty

breathing pattern

    biot

    Cheyne-Stokes

    eupneic

    Kussmaul

    shallow

    tachypneic

cachectic

cachexia

comatose

cushingoid

cyanosis

cyanotic

diaphoresis

diaphoretic

disheveled

dyspnea

dyspneic

emaciated

flat affect

halitosis

lethargic

listless

mask facies

mask-like facies

neat and well groomed

no acute distress

nontoxic-appearing

obtunded

oriented to person, place, and time

orthostatic changes

pallor

speech

    babbling

    dysarthric

    garbled

    halting

    jerky

    lisping

    muttered

    monotonous

    pressured

    rapid

    slurred

    stuttering

stertorous

stridorous

tachypnea

tachypneic

well-developed

well-nourished

TERMS RELATED TO VITAL SIGNS

afebrile, febrile

blood pressure 120/80 mmHg (millimeters of mercury)

height

oxygen (O_2) saturation

pulse rate 80/minute

respiratory rate 18/minute (labored, unlabored)

temperature 98.6 degrees (Tmax = temperature maximum)

weight

TERMS RELATED TO THE SKIN

abrasions

acne

cherry angiomata

clammy

complexion

    ashen

    flushed

    jaundice

    pale

    pallid

    pallor

    ruddy

    sallow

ecchymosis; ecchymoses (plural)

ecchymotic

eczema

eczematoid

eczematous

edematous

erythema

erythematosus

herpes simplex

herpes zoster

herpetic lesions

lichenoid edema

maculopapular rash

maculopapule

malar rash

petechiae

plethoric

purpura

seborrhea/seborrheic keratosis

spider angiomata

stigmata of liver disease

telangiectasis

tenting (skin, tissue)

tinea cruris

turgor

ulcer

urticaria

varicella

vermillion border or lesion

verrucous lesion

vesicle/vesicular

vitiligo

warm and dry

welts

wheals

TERMS RELATED TO HEENT

Head

alopecia

anterior fontanelle (baby examination)

atraumatic

atraumatic, normocephalic (AT, NA)

Battle sign

cephalohematoma

dandruff

flattening of the (left, right) nasolabial fold

fontanelle

macrocephalic

macrocephaly

male-pattern baldness

megacephalic

megacephaly

nasolabial fold

normocephalic

occiput

tinea capitis

torticollis

Eyes

amblyopia

anicteric

anterior chamber

arcus senilis

arterial pulsation

arteriolar narrowing

arteriovenous (AV) nicking

astigmatism

best-corrected visual acuity

blepharitis

blown pupil

cataract

chalazion

conjunctiva (plural conjunctivae)

conjunctival hemorrhage/injection

conjunctivitis

cornea clear/cloudy

corneal abrasion

corneal opacity

corneal reflex intact

cross-eyed

diabetic retinopathy

disk margins well delineated

disks sharp

enucleated

exophthalmos

extraocular movements intact (EOMI)

exudate

farsightedness

flame hemorrhages

fluorescein stain

foreign body

fundi well visualized, not well visualized, not examined

fundus

funduscopic examination

funduscopy

glaucoma

hemorrhage or exudate (H or E)

homonymous hemianopsia

hordeolum

icterus

iridectomy

iritis

isocoria

isocoric

Kayser-Fleischer ring

Keith-Wagener changes

LASIK surgery

lens implantation

lenticular opacification

lid lag

macular degeneration

Marcus Gunn pupil

myopia

narrow-angle glaucoma

nearsightedness

nystagmus

oblique muscle

OD (right eye)

opacification

opacified

ophthalmoplegia

optic nerve

OS (left eye)

OU (both eyes)

pallor disks

papilledema

periorbital edema

peripheral vision

pinguecula

pink eye

presbyopia

pterygium

ptosis (dictated as TOH-SIS)

pupils (fixed/dilated/pinpoint)

pupils equal and reactive to light (PERL)

pupils equal, round, and reactive to light and accommodation (PERRLA)

pupils equal, round, and reactive to light (PERRL)

raccoon eyes

rapid eye movements (REM)

rectus muscle

red reflex

retinopathy

Roth spots

rust ring

sclerae anicteric/icteric/nonicteric

silver wire effect

slit lamp

small blot hemorrhages

strabismus

visual acuity

wide-angle glaucoma

Wood's lamp/light

Ears

acoustic neuroma

AD (right ear)

air bone gap

AS (left ear)

AU (both ears)

audiogram

auditory canal

auditory discrimination

auditory threshold

auditory tube

barotitis

bulging tympanic membranes

calorie test

cerumen

cholesteatoma

cochlea

cochlea implant

conductive hearing loss

deafness

decibels

Dix-Hallpike test

dysequilibrium

eardrum

equilibrium

eustachian tube

external ear

finger rub test

hearing impairment

hemotympanum

hertz

impacted cerumen

injected tympanic membrane

injection

labyrinthitis

middle ear

myringitis

myringotomy tubes

nasoseptoplasty

neurosensory hearing loss

otitis media externa

otorrhea

PE tube (polyethylene tube)

perforation

pinna

pneumoscopic exam

presbycusis

Rinne test

serous fluid

tympanic membranes (TMs)

vertigo

vestibular disease/function

vibrating fork

Weber test

Nose

airway obstruction

congested

flattening of the nasolabial fold

inferior turbinate

nares (plural naris)

nasolabial fold

polyp

postnasal drip

septal deviation

septoplasty

turbinate hypertrophy

Mouth and Throat (Oral Examination)

aphthae

aphthous ulcers

base of tongue

beefy red tonsils

buccal mucosa

canker sore

cleft palate

cobblestoning

dentition

edentulous

erythema

exudate

gag reflex

geographic tongue

gingivae

gingivitis

globus hystericus

glossitis

hard palate

leukoplakia

mucopus

mucous membranes moist/dry

palate

peritonsillar abscess

pharyngeal wall

pharyngopalatine

pharynx

protruded tongue midline

soft palate

temporomandibular joint

thrush

tonsillar hypertrophy

uvula moves on phonation

uvula and tongue midline

TERMS RELATED TO THE NECK

carotid bruit

cervical adenopathy

cervical chain

cervical lymphadenopathy

goiter

hepatojugular reflux (HJR)

jugular venous distention (JVD)

lymph nodes nonpalpable/palpable

lymphadenopathy

multinodular goiter

nuchal rigidity

pharynx

shotty lymph nodes

supple

thyroid nodule

thyroid nonpalpable

thyromegaly

trachea midline

tracheal deviation

venous distention at 45 degrees

TERMS RELATED TO THE CHEST AND BREASTS

AP diameter (anteroposterior diameter)

areola

atrophic

axilla

barrel chest

breasts atrophic

colostrum

costal margins

costochondritis

fissuring of the nipple

funnel chest

galactorrhea

glands of Montgomery

gynecomastia

hollow chest

intercostal space

inverted nipple

mastectomy

no lumps or masses

no nipple discharge

peau d'orange

pectus carinatum

pectus excavatum

permanent pacemaker

pigeon breast

precordium quiet

status post mastectomy

sternoclavicular joint

sternocostal joint

sternotomy scar

sternum

supramammary nipple

suprasternal notch

suprasternal retractions

Tanner

thoracic

thorax

xiphoid

TERMS RELATED TO THE LUNGS

absent breath sounds

accessory muscles of respiration

adventitious breath sounds

AP (auscultation and percussion)

AP diameter normal/increased

apex

apical area

atelectasis

bibasilar rales

bronchial asthma

bronchophony

bronchoscopy

bronchospasm

bronchovesicular

clear to auscultation and percussion (A & P or P & A)

coarse friction rub

coarse rales/rhonchi

consolidation

costophrenic angles

cough

    bubbling

    croupy

    hacking

    harsh

    hollow

    loose

    nonproductive

    productive

    rasping

    rattling

    wracking

Cheyne-Stokes breathing

collapsed lung

crepitant rales

crepitus

decreased breath sounds

dullness to percussion

dyspnea

dyspnea on exertion

dyspneic

egophony

empyema

end-expiratory wheeze

expiration

expiratory time (normal/pronounced)

expiratory wheeze

forced expiratory time

fremitus

friction rub

grating friction rub

harsh friction rub

hemidiaphragm

hemothorax

hyperresonant

hyperventilation

hyporesonant

hypoventilation

inspiration

inspiratory wheeze

lung fields

moist rales

muffled breath sounds

percussion

pleural rub

rales

resonant

rhonchi

rub

unlabored breathing, without retractions or grunting

wheeze

whispered pectoriloquy

TERMS RELATED TO THE HEART

1st and 2nd heart sounds are normal; no 3rd or 4th heart sound heard. Type *S1 & S2 normal; no S3 or S4 heard*.

A2 louder than P2

accentuated heart sound

aortic click

aortic regurgitation

apical systolic murmur

arrhythmias

asystole

atrial fibrillation (often dictated as A-Fib or AF)

atrial flutter

bradycardia

bruit

click

ejection fraction

gallop

grade I/6, 2/6, 3/6, 4/6, 5/6

grade I, grade II, grade IV, grade V, grade VI

heart sound

heave

holosystolic murmur

intercostal space

irregularly/irregular

knock

midclavicular line

mitral valve prolapse

mitral valve regurgitation

multifocal atrial tachycardia (MAT)

murmur

> crescendo
>
> decrescendo
>
> diastolic
>
> diminuendo
>
> ejection
>
> systolic

murmur radiating to the axilla or neck

normal sinus rhythm (NSR)

P2 louder than A2

parasternal border

pericardial knock

physiologically split

point of maximal impulse (PMI) in the 5th intercostal space

premature ventricular contraction (PVC)

prosthetic click/sound

rapid ventricular response

regular rate and rhythm (RRR)

regular sinus rhythm (RSR)

regurgitation

rub

S1, S2, S3, S4 (heart sounds 1, 2, 3, & 4)

S1 equals S2

S1 and S2 normal, no S3 or S4

S3 gallop

supraventricular tachycardia (SVT)

systolic ejection murmur

tachycardia

thrill

tricuspid valve

TERMS RELATED TO THE ABDOMEN

acute abdomen

ascites

auscultation

ballotable

bowel sounds normal, normoactive, hyperactive, hypoactive, high-pitched, inaudible, tympanitic, decreased, diminished

bruit

costovertebral

direct hernia

distended

exogenous obesity

femoral hernia

fluid wave

guarding

hernia

    direct

    incarcerated

    indirect

    inguinal

    strangulated

hyperresonant

landmarks

    axillary line

    costophrenic angle

    costovertebral angle

    epigastric

    inguinal

    left costal margin

    left lower quadrant

    left upper quadrant

    ligament of Treitz

    McBurney's point

    midclavicular line

    Murphy's point

    paramedian

    parasternal border

    right costal margin

    right lower quadrant

    right upper quadrant

    suprapubic area

    xiphoid to pubis

liver and spleen

    1-2 fingerbreadths below the right costal margin

    hepatosplenomegaly

    liver, spleen, and kidneys enlarged/nonpalpable/not felt

    organomegaly

    tender, nontender

morbid obesity

obese

omental apron

organomegaly

palpable, nonpalpable

panniculus

percussion

peristaltic activity

Pfannenstiel incision

protuberant

rebound

rebound tenderness

Rovsing's sign

scaphoid

scars of previous surgery

silent abdomen

tender, nontender

tympanitic

vascular

visceromegaly

xiphoid process

TERMS RELATED TO THE BACK

cauda equina

cervical spine (C-spine)

costovertebral angle tenderness (CVA)

dextroscoliosis

dorsal spine

dorsokyphosis

hump back

kyphosis

levoscoliosis

lordosis

lumbar spine (L-spine)

lumbosacral

palpation

paravertebral

point tenderness

radiation

referred pain

rotoscoliosis

sacrum

sciatic notch

sciatica

scoliosis

spina bifida

spinal column

spine

supraspinatus

thoracic spine (T-spine)

vertebral column

TERMS RELATED TO THE EXTREMITIES

abduction

AC joint (acromioclavicular)

Ace bandage

adduction

AKA (above-knee amputation)

Apley test

arthroplasty

atrophy

avulsion fracture

Baker cyst

BKA (below-knee amputation)

Bouchard nodes

boutonniere deformity

brawny edema

buffalo hump

bunion

calf tenderness

capillary refill

carpal tunnel syndrome

claudication

clicking

clubbing

cockup splint

cords

coronoid process

coxa valga

coxa vara

crepitus

cyanosis, clubbing, or edema (CCE)

de Quervain tendinitis

decubitus ulcer

dependent edema

DIP (distal interphalangeal) joint

Doppler

dorsalis pedal (DP) pulses

dorsalis pedis pulse

dorsiflexion

dowager's hump

drawer sign

edema (1+, 2+, or 3+)

edematous

femoral pulse

fibromyalgia

Finklestein's test

full range of motion

hallux valgus deformity

Heberden's nodes

hemarthrosis

hip click (baby examination)

Homans' sign

Lachman's sign (dictated as "lockman")

laxity

leg length discrepancy

ligament

lupus erythematosus

McMurray's test

MCP (metacarpophalangeal) joint

Mills

mottling

myofibrositis

myositis

navicular fracture

Neer 90/90

nursemaid elbow

onychia

paronychia

pedal edema

perionychia/perionychium

peripheral pulses

PIP (proximal interphalangeal) joint

pitting edema

plantar fasciitis

polyarthralgia

polyarthropathy

polymyalgia rheumatica

popliteal pulse

posterior tibial pulses (PT)

pulses 2+ and equal bilaterally

quadriceps

range of motion

rotator cuff

sacroiliac joints

saphenous vein

sciatic notch

sciatica

snuffbox

stress test

styloid process

swan-neck deformity

tendon

tennis elbow

thenar eminence

thoracic outlet syndrome

Tinel test

torticollis

trigger finger

trigger point

trochanter (greater/lesser)

ulnar distribution

valgus deformity

valgus stress

varicose veins

varicosities

varus test

vascular compromise

venous stasis

wryneck

Yergason test

TERMS RELATED TO THE RECTUM

ampulla

anal prolapse/protrusion

anal verge

anoderm

benign prostatic hypertrophy (BPH)

fecal impaction

fissure

fistula in ano

guaiac positive/negative stool

heme positive/negative stool

Hemoccult positive/negative

hemorrhoid

hemorrhoidal tags

internal hemorrhoid

melena

occult blood

perineum

pouch

prostate enlarged/boggy/tender

prostatic hypertrophy

sentinel pile

sigmoidoscopy

sphincter tone

tarry stool

thrombosed hemorrhoid

vault empty

TERMS RELATED TO THE GENITOURINARY TRACT AND PELVIS

adnexa

anteverted uterus

bimanual exam

Braxton-Hicks contractions

breech presentation

BSU (Bartholin, Skene, and urethral glands)

cephalic presentation

Chadwick's sign

chordee

circumcised

cul-de-sac

dyspareunia

effaced

EGBUS: external genitalia and Bartholin, urethral, and Skene glands

epididymis

epididymitis

female escutcheon

fetal heart tones (FHTs)

glans penis

herpes

herpes zoster

herpetic lesions

intact hymen

Kegel exercises

labia

lochia

marital introitus

menarche

mittelschmerz

monilia

mons pubis

normal for age

normal male/female genitalia

normal postmenopausal

nulliparous

ovarian cyst

palpable mass

Pap smear

parous

pediculus pubis

pelvic examination

perineal

perineum

phimosis

pregnant uterus, 6 weeks' size

rectovaginal exam

scrotum

speculum

status post orchiectomy

Tanner growth chart

Tanner stage I, II, III, etc.

testes descended

testicular torsion

tocolysis

transverse lie

urethral caruncle

urethral meatus

uterine prolapse

uterus anteverted

vaginocele

vagina

vaginal discharge

vaginal rugae

vaginal vault

venereal warts

verruca acuminatum

vestibulitis

vulva

TERMS RELATED TO NEUROLOGICAL CONDITIONS

ankle jerks

aphagia

aphasia

ataxia

Babinski (downgoing/upgoing)

Bell palsy

cerebellar

cogwheel rigidity

confrontation

coordination

corneal reflex/response

cranial nerves 2–12 grossly intact

deep tendon reflexes (DTRs)

diabetic neuropathy of the feet

doll's eye reflex/sign

dysdiadochokinesias

extrapyramidal

face symmetric

facial strength and sensation

familial tremors

finger-to-nose testing

flattening of the nasolabial fold

flexors downgoing

gag reflex

gait
    ataxic
    antalgic
    apraxic
    athetotic
    broad-based
    dystonic
    festination
    glue-footed
    hemiplegic
    hysterical
    scissors
    shuffling
    spastic
    staggering
    Trendelenburg
    waddling
    wide-based
gait and station
gaze preference
Hallpike maneuver
heel-to-shin test
hemiparesis
hemiplegia
Homans' sign
homonymous field defect
homonymous hemianopsia
Hunt/Hess classification III
intention tremor
knee jerk
Lasegue test
Marfan syndrome
meningeal sign
Moro's sign/reflex
Moses
motor power
motor or sensory deficits

neuralgia

nonfocal

noxious stimulation

nystagmus

oculocephalic maneuver

paresthesias

Phalen's sign

pill-rolling tremors

pinprick/pinwheel

plantar flexion

plantar reflexes (downgoing/upgoing/equivocal/withdrawal)

polyneuritis

posturing

proprioception

rapid alternating movements

reflexes

  achilles

  biceps

  brachioradialis

  Chaddock

  Gordon

  grasp

  Hoffman

  Mayer

  Oppenheim

  quadriceps

  triceps

  Wartenberg

Romberg's sign

sensory deficit/loss

sign

  Brudzinski

  Glabellar

  Kernig

  Myerson

  Stewart-Holmes

  Trousseau

speech (fluent, dysarthric)

station

stereognosis

stocking distribution

straight leg raising position/negative at 45 degrees

strength and sensation intact

stuporous

suck and grasp

tandem walk

temperative sense

tic

Tinel's sign

titubation (head or trunk tremor)

tongue protrudes in the midline

two-point discrimination

vibratory sense

visual fields are full

TERMS RELATED TO MENTAL STATUS

ADD (attention deficit disorder)

affect (appropriate/flat)

agoraphobia

alert and oriented ×3 (person, place, and time)

amnesia

autistic

axis I: clinical disorders, syndromes, and other areas of concern

axis II: personality disorders and mental retardation

axis III: medical conditions (which may impact emotions)

axis IV: psychosocial stressors (e.g., death, divorce, loss of job)

axis V: global assessment of functioning

bipolar disorder

claustrophobia

decision making

delusions

depression

flat affect

flight of ideas

hallucinations

hyperactive/hypoactive

ideas of reference

low self-esteem

manic depressive disorder

narcissism

obsessive-compulsive disorder (OCD)

paranoid schizophrenia

phobia

psychosocial stressors

sensorium

short attention span

suicidal ideations

tests

    BNMSE (Brief Neuropsychological Mental Status)

    GOAT (Galveston Orientation & Amnesia Test)

    Goodenough Draw-A-Man

    Halsted-Wepman Aphasia Screening

    MMPI (Minnesota Multiphasic Personality Inventory)

    Porteus Maze Test

    Rorschach Test

    Stanford-Binet Intelligence

    WAIS (Wechsler Adult Intelligence Scale)

    Wechsler Memory Scale

    Zung

Body Systems

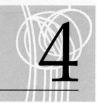

CARDIOVASCULAR SYSTEM

2-, 3-, 4-vessel bypass/disease

4-chamber view

ACE inhibitor

adenosine

ambulatory monitor

anemia

angina

angina pectoris

angioplasty

anterior descending

anticoagulation

aorta

aortic cusp

aortic outflow murmur

aortic stenosis

aortic valve

arrhythmia

arteriosclerotic

ASCVD (arteriosclerotic cardiovascular disease)

atherosclerosis

atrial fibrillation

atrioseptal

atrium

AV node ablation

beta blocker

Betapace

Biotronik

bradycardia

Bruce protocol

bruit

CABG (coronary artery bypass grafting)

cardiac enzymes

cardiac isoenzymes

Cardiolite scan

cardiomegaly

cardioversion

Cardizem CD

carotid artery

catheterization

cauterized

Chiari complex (sounds like QRA complex)

cholesterol

circumflex

color-flow Doppler

congenital heart defect

congestive heart failure

continuous color flow

cor pulmonale

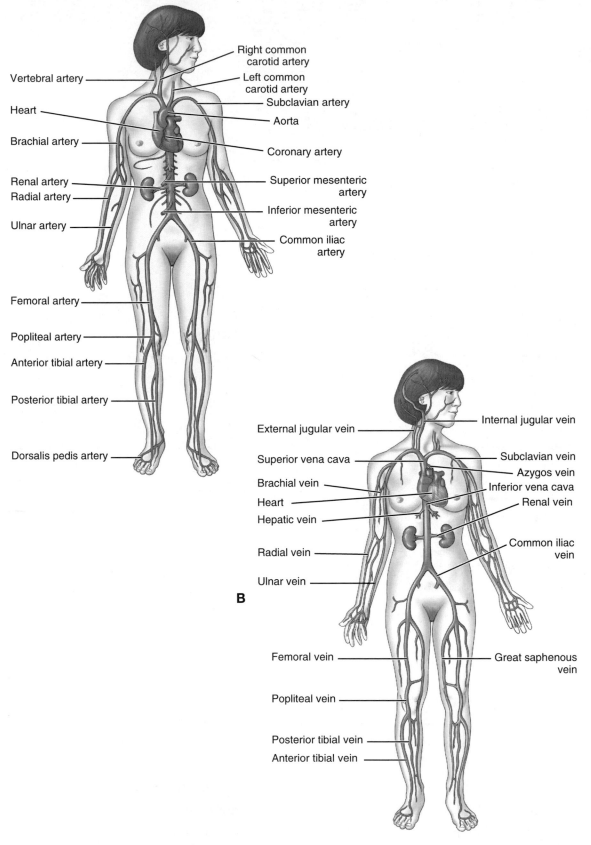

FIGURE **4-1** The circulatory system. **A,** Arteries. **B,** Veins. (Modified from Brown JL: *Medical insurance made easy,* Philadelphia, 2001, WB Saunders.)

coronary angiography

coronary artery bypass

Coumadin

deep vein thrombosis

defibrillation

diuretic/diuresed/diuresis

dobutamine

Doppler study

dorsalis pedis pulses

double product

dyslipidemia

dysrhythmia

E:A (dictated as E to A)

ECG (electrocardiogram)

echocardiogram (ECHO)

echocardiography

ectopy/ectopics

EF (ejection fraction)

ejection fraction

EKG (electrocardiogram)

electrocardioversion

endarterectomy

endocardial

endocardium

EP study (electrophysiologic study)

event monitor (30 days)

fascicular heart block

fasciculation

femoral pulses

furosemide

gallop

gated scan

HDL (high-density lipids)

HDL cholesterol

heparin

hepatic

Holter monitor (24-hr)

hydrochlorothiazide

hypercholesterolemia

hypertension (controlled)

implantation

infarction

INR (international normal rate)

interrogation

isoenzyme

J point depression

King of Hearts Monitor

LAD (left anterior descending)

Lanoxin

Lasix

LC possible

LDL (low-density lipids)

LDL cholesterol

LIMA graft (left internal mammary artery)

lipid panel

Lipitor

liver function panel/studies/test

mammary graft

Medcast

Medtronic

MI (myocardial infarction)

mid left anterior

mitral insufficiency

mitral regurgitation

mitral valve prolapse

M-mode

MPHR (maximum predicted heart rate)

MUGA scan

murmur

myocardial infarction

myocardium

NIR Primo stent (sounds like near)

NIR Royale stent

ostial

P, Q, R, S, T, waves

paced rhythm

pacemaker

palpitations

paroxysmal atrial contractions

paroxysmal atrial tachycardia

peripheral pulses

Persantine

Phizer

physiologically split

PMI (point of maximum impulse)

porcine valve

posterior tibial

Primo stent

Prince of Hearts Monitor

procainamide

prosthetic valve

proximal

PT (prothrombin time)

PTCA (percutaneous transluminal coronary angioplasty)

PTT (partial thromboplastin time)

pulmonary valve

pulmonary vein

pulse wave

QDS

QRS wave/depression

radial pulses

radioablation

rub

S1, S2, S3, S4

St. Jude valve

saphenous vein graft

scintigraphy

Sestamibi scan

sick sinus syndrome

SPECT

ST segment depression

stenosis

stent

ST-T depression/elevation

subendocardial infarction

tachybrady syndrome

tachycardia

TEE (transesophageal echocardiography)

telemetry

thallium treadmill

thromboembolism

thrombophlebitis

thrombosis

TPA

tricuspid valve

trileaflet

troponin I level

T-wave alternans

upsloping

ventricular

ventricular pacing

Viagra

VLDL

VVI pacing

wall motion abnormality

Cardiac Heart Failure Classification

Class I: asymptomatic

Class II: comfortable at rest, symptomatic with normal activity

Class III: comfortable at rest, symptomatic with less than normal activity

Class IV: severe cardiac failure

Electrocardiogram (EKG or ECG)

1. For **standard bipolar leads,** use Roman numerals. EXAMPLE: lead I, lead II, lead III.

2. For **augmented limb leads,** use a lowercase *a,* followed by an uppercase *V,* followed by an uppercase *R* (right), *L* (left), or *F* (front). EXAMPLE: aVR, aVL, aVF.

3. For **precordial limb leads,** enter the numeral in the same point size on-line with the V, with no space between. EXAMPLE: V1, V2, V3, V4, V5, V6, V7, V8, V9.

4. Enter the numeral in the same point size on-line with the V, with no space between. EXAMPLE: V3R, V4R.

5. For **Ensiform cardiac leads,** enter E in the same point size on-line with the V, with no space between. EXAMPLE: VE.

Tracing Terms

J junction

J point

P wave

PR interval

Q wave

QRS interval, prolongation, etc.

QS wave

QT interval, prolongation, etc.

R wave

S wave

ST segment, depression, etc.

ST-T segment, elevation, etc.

T wave

Ta wave

U wave

Pacemaker Codes

Capitalize these three-letter codes without spaces or periods. EXAMPLE: AVD.

First and second letters refer to the following:

A   atrium

V   ventricle

D   both atrium and ventricle

O   neither atrium nor ventricle

Third letter refers to the following:

I   inhibited response

T   triggered response

D   inhibited and triggered response

O   no response

DICTATED: A grade four over six murmur is noted.

TYPE: A grade 4/6 murmur is noted.

Murmur Names

ASM   atrial systolic murmur

CM   continuous murmur

DM   diastolic murmur

DSM   delayed systolic murmur

ESM   ejection systolic murmur

IDM   immediate diastolic murmur

LSM   late systolic murmur

PSM   pansystolic murmur

SDM   systolic-diastolic murmur

SEM   systolic ejection murmur

SM   systolic murmur

Murmur Grades

Grade 1:   barely audible

Grade 2:   quiet, but clearly audible

Grade 3:   moderately loud

Grade 4:   loud

Grade 5:   very loud; audible with stethoscope partly off the chest

Grade 6:   so loud that it can be heard with stethoscope just above the chest wall

Bruits

AEC   aortic ejection click
AOC   aortic opening click
C   click
E   ejection sound
EC   ejection click
NEC   nonejection click
OS   opening snap
PEC   pulmonary ejection click
SC   systolic click
SS   summation sound
W   whoop

Heart Sounds

S1   first heart sound
S2   second heart sound
S3   third heart sound
S4   fourth heart sound

DICTATED: Normal first and second heart sounds.

TYPE: Normal S1 and S2.

DIGESTIVE SYSTEM

acute abdominal series

alcoholism

anorexia

appendicitis

barium swallow

Barrett's esophagitis

BE/barium enema

belch

borborygmi

bright red blood

bright red blood per rectum

cholecystectomy

cholecystitis

choledocholithiasis

cholelithiasis

cirrhosis

CLO test

Clostridium difficile (C. difficile)

colic

colitis

colonoscopy

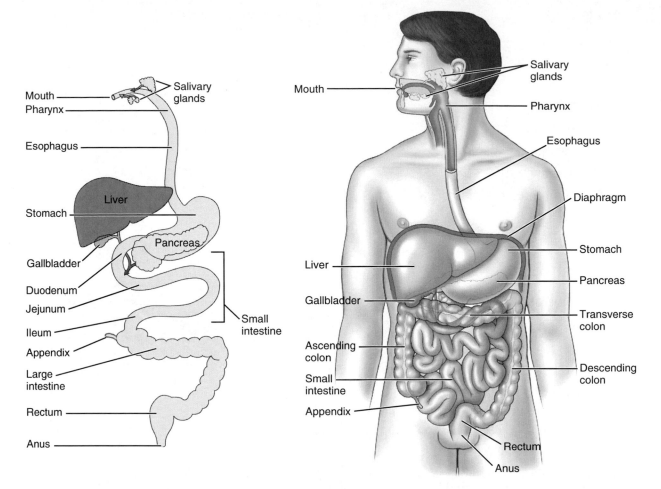

FIGURE **4-2** The digestive system. (Modified from Brown JL: *Medical insurance made easy,* Philadelphia, 2001, WB Saunders.)

constipation

Crohn disease

DeMeester score/scale

diarrhea

digital exam

diverticulitis

diverticulum

duodenum

dyspepsia

dysphagia

early satiety

emesis

endoscopy

enterocolitis

esophagitis

flat plate of the abdomen

flatulence

flatus

flexible sigmoidoscopy

gallbladder

gastric bypass/resection

gastritis

gastroenteritis

guaiac positive/negative

Helicobacter pylori (H. pylori)
hematemesis
hematochezia
heme negative/positive
Hemoccult positive/negative
hepatitis

icterus
ileostomy
ileum/ileus
inflammatory bowel disease
irritable bowel syndrome

jaundice

laparoscopy
laparotomy

malabsorption
Mallory-Weiss tear/syndrome

obstipation
odynophagia

pancreatitis
plain film
polyp
postprandial
pyloric

rebound tenderness
reflux
regurgitate
rotavirus

sphincter tone
splenomegaly
steatorrhea
stricture

tarry stools

ulcerative colitis
ultrasound
upper GI series

volvulus

Food-Borne Illnesses
Bacteria
Bacillus cereus
Brucella

Campylobacter jejuni
Clostridium botulinum
Clostridium perfringens

Escherichia coli

Leptospira interrogans
Listeria monocytogenes

Salmonella
Shigella
Staphylococcus aureus
streptococcus group A

Vibrio cholerae/parahaemolyticus

Yersinia enterocolitica

Fish/Shellfish
ciguatera

neurotoxic shellfish

paralytic shellfish

scombroid

Heavy Metals
arsenic

cadmium
copper

mercury
monosodium glutamate

niacin

tin

zinc

Parasites
Anisakis
Ascaris lumbricoides

Cryptosporidium
Cyclospora

Diphyllobothrium latum

Entamoeba histolytica

Giardia lamblia

Taenia species
Trichinella spiralis

Miscellaneous
Brainerd diarrhea

mushroom

Varian Creutzfeldt-Jakob disease

ENDOCRINE SYSTEM

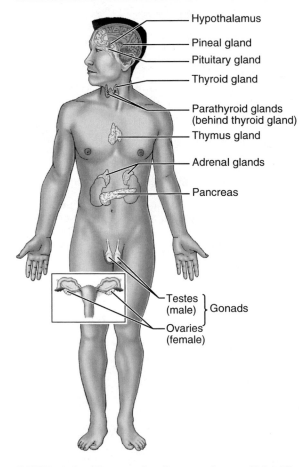

- Hypothalamus
- Pineal gland
- Pituitary gland
- Thyroid gland
- Parathyroid glands (behind thyroid gland)
- Thymus gland
- Adrenal glands
- Pancreas
- Testes (male)
- Ovaries (female)
- Gonads

FIGURE **4-3** The endocrine system. (Modified from Brown JL: *Medical insurance made easy,* Philadelphia, 2001, WB Saunders.)

Accu-Chek
Accu-Chek Advance
adrenal

choice needle-free insulin injector

euthyroid
exophthalmus

Glucometer Elite blood glucose monitor
glucose
glycosuria
goiter
Graves' disease

Hashimoto's thyroiditis
hyperthyroidism
hypothyroidism

islets of Langerhans

One Touch diabetes test strip

parathyroid
polydipsia

polyphagia

polyuria

Precision QI-D meter

proteinuria

stasis ulcer

thyroiditis

thyromegaly

thyrotoxicosis

INTEGUMENTARY SYSTEM

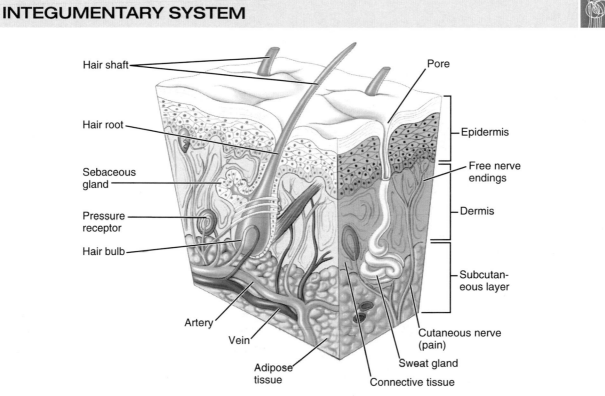

FIGURE **4-4**   The skin. (Modified from Brown JL: *Medical insurance made easy,* Philadelphia, 2001, WB Saunders.)

abrasion

abscess

acne

acne vulgaris

actinic cheilitis

actinic keratosis

actinomycosis

alopecia

athlete's foot

basal cell carcinoma

blister

boil

carcinoma

cellulitis

comedone

contusion

coxsackie virus

cyst

dermatitis

dermatomyositis

ecchymosis

eczema

epithelium, epithelial

eruption

erythema

eschar

excoriation

fever blister

fissure

fluctuant

fungal infection

furuncle

hand-foot-mouth disease

herpes

hirsutism

hives

impetigo

indurated

intertrigo

keloid

laceration

lesion

maculae

maculopapular rash

melanoma

Mohs' surgery

mole

nevi, nevus

nodule

papule

pediculosis

plantar

pustule

radiodermatitis

rhus dermatitis

scabies

seborrhea

seborrheic

squamous cell

verruca

vesicle

vesicular

vitiligo

vulgaris

welts

wheal

MUSCULOSKELETAL SYSTEM

acetabulum

acromial

alignment

ankylosing spondylitis

antalgic

Apley grind/scratch test

apprehension

arthralgia

arthritis

arthroscopy

avulsion

Baker's cyst

Buck's traction

buddy tape

bursitis

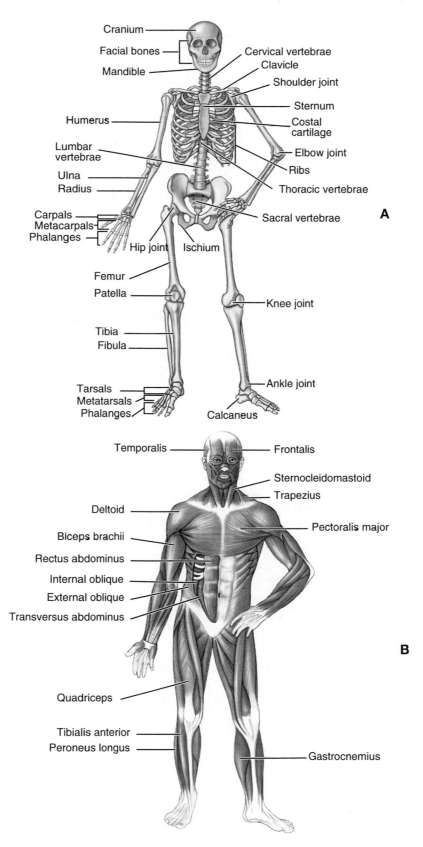

FIGURE **4-5**   The musculoskeletal system. **A,** Skeleton. **B,** Muscles. (Modified from Brown JL: *Medical insurance made easy,* Philadelphia, 2001, WB Saunders.)

carpal tunnel syndrome

cauda equina

Charcot's joint

chondrosis

Codman exercises

Colles' fracture

costochondritis

Cozen sign

crepitus

C-spine (cervical spine)

degenerative joint disease

DEXA scan (bone density)

diaphysial

diaphysis

dislocation

DJD (degenerative joint disease)

drawer sign

DTRs (deep tendon reflexes)

effusion

EMG (electromyelogram)

ENDOPEARL (used in ligament repair)

epiphyseal growth plate

facet

fascia lata

fibromyalgia

foramen

Fosamax

Garre's osteomyelitis

gout/gouty arthritis

heel-and-toe walk

herniated disk

HNP (herniated nucleus pulposus)

impingement test

intertrochanteric

Lachman's test

laminectomy

lateral facets

ligamentum flavum

lupus

McMurray's test

Merchant's view

myoglobin

myoglobinemia

myositis

Osgood-Schlatter

osteoarthritis

osteopenia

osteophytes

paravertebral

paresthesia

Patrick's test

Phalen test

polyarthritis

prosthesis

radiculopathy

range-of-motion test

rhabdomyolysis

sciatica

spring test

straight leg raise test

subluxation

tendinitis

tennis elbow

TENS unit

Tinel's sign

Muscles

Achilles tendon

biceps brachii

biceps femoris (hamstring)

deltoid

external oblique

frontalis

gastrocnemius
gluteus maximus

latissimus dorsi

occipitalis

pectoralis major

rectus abdominis
rectus femoris (quadriceps)

sartorius
serratus anterior
sternocleidomastoid

tibialis anterior
trapezius
triceps

vastus medialls

Skeletal Bones
calcaneus (heel)
carpals (wrist)
cervical vertebra (neck)
clavicle
coccyx
cranium

elbow

femur
fibula
frontal bone

greater trochanter

humerus

iliac crest
ilium (hip)

mandible
mastoid process
maxilla
metacarpals (hand)
metatarsals (foot)

occipital bone
orbit

parietal bone
patella (kneecap)
pelvic girdle
phalanges (fingers/toes)

radius
ribs

sacrum
scapula (shoulder blade)
sternum
symphysis pubis

tarsal (ankle)
temporal bone
tibia

ulna

xiphoid process

zygomatic arch

Spine
cervical
lumbar
thoracic

NERVOUS SYSTEM AND PSYCHIATRY

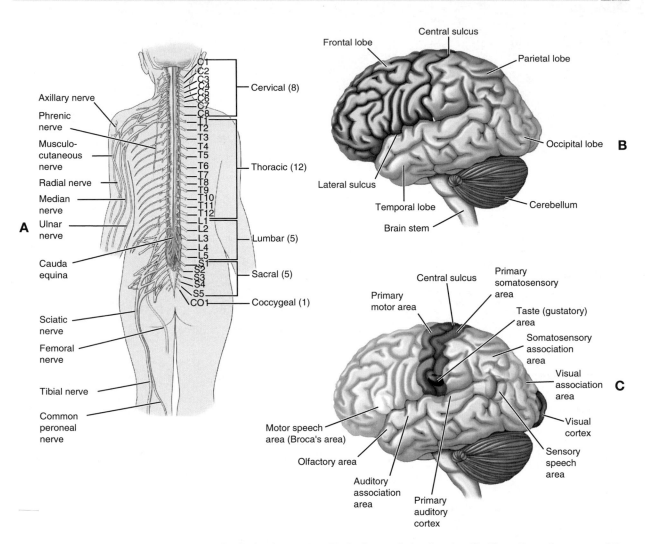

FIGURE **4-6** The nervous system. **A,** Spinal nerves. **B,** Lobes of the brain. **C,** Functional areas of the brain. (Modified from Brown JL: *Medical insurance made easy,* Philadelphia, 2001, WB Saunders.)

abuse

ADD (attention deficit disorder)

addiction

alcoholism

Alzheimer disease

amyotrophic lateral sclerosis

anorexia nervosa

anxiety

aphasia

apraxia

ataxia

auditory hallucinations

bipolar disorder

BNMSE (Brief Neuropsychological Mental Status Examination)

Brudzinski's sign
bulimia nervosa

cerebrovascular accident
clinical depression
concussion
confusion

depression
diabetic neuropathy
disorientation
DTRs (deep tendon reflexes)
dysphasia

eating disorder
EEG (electroencephalogram)
encephalopathy

finger-nose test
focal

GOAT (Galveston Orientation and Amnesia
   Test)

Hallpike maneuver
hallucination
Hunt/Hess classification
hydrocephalus
hysteria

insomnia
insomnolence

labyrinthitis
lightheadedness
Lou Gehrig disease

mental disorder
migraine
MMPI (Minnesota Multiphasic Personality
   Inventory)

mood swings
Moses
motor strength
MRI (magnetic resonance imaging)
multiple sclerosis

nervous disorder
neurogenic claudication
neurosis
nuchal rigidity
numbness
nystagmus

OCD (obsessive-compulsive disorder)

panic attacks
paralysis
paresthesia
Parkinson disease
photophobia
psychiatric
psychology
psychosis
psychotic
ptosis

Revised Trauma Score

schizophrenia
sciatica
suicidal ideation
syncope

Tabes neuropathy
TENS unit
TIA (transient ischemic attack)
tic
Tinel's sign

vertigo
visual hallucinations

Seizures

absence seizure

atonic seizure

clonic seizure

complex partial seizure

convulsive seizure

cryptogenic epilepsy

focal seizure

generalized onset seizure

grand mal seizure

idiopathic seizure

jacksonian seizure

myoclonic epilepsy

nonconvulsive seizure

partial seizure

petit mal seizure

pseudoseizure

psychomotor seizure

status epilepticus

temporal lobe seizure

tonic seizure

tonic-clonic seizure

EEG

alpha rhythm

beta rhythm

brain waves

dysrhythmia

Glasgow Coma Scale (GCS)

Eye Opening (E)

4 = Spontaneous

3 = To voice

2 = To pain

1 = None

Motor Response (M)

6 = Normal

5 = Localizes to pain

4 = Withdraws to pain

3 = Decorticate posture

2 = Decerebrate

1 = None

Example: E4 V5 M6

Example: E2 Vintubated M5

Verbal Response (V)

5 = Normal conversation

4 = Disoriented conversation

3 = Words, but not coherent

2 = No words; only sounds

1 = None

Vintubated = intubated patient

REPRODUCTIVE SYSTEM

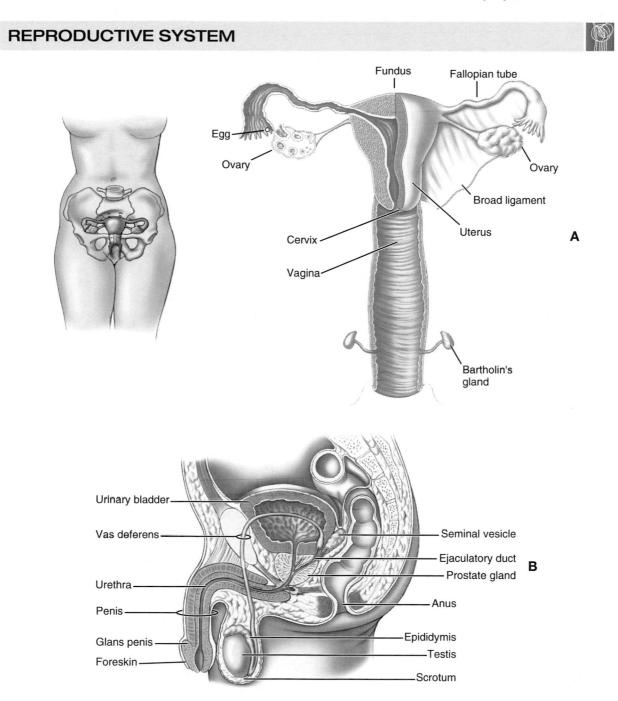

FIGURE **4-7** The reproductive system. **A,** Female. **B,** Male. (Modified from Brown JL: *Medical insurance made easy,* Philadelphia, 2001, WB Saunders.)

AIDS

amenorrhea

anorgasmia

Apgar score

bacterial vaginosis

Bartholin gland

BSO (bilateral salpingo-oophorectomy)

CA (cancer)

Candida

cervical os

cervicitis

cervix nonfriable

Chandlelier sign

Chlamydia

circumcision

clue cells

coitus interruptus

colposcopy

condyloma

cryotherapy

cystic breast disease

cystorrhaphy

dysmenorrhea

dyspareunia

dysplasia

efflux

ejaculate

ejaculation

endocervical curettage

endometriosis

epididymitis

erectile dysfunction

erosion

eversion

GC (gonorrhea)

GEN probe

gynecomastia

herpes

HIV (human immunodeficiency virus)

HPV (human papillomavirus)

hysterectomy

induration

introitus

Kegel exercises

KOH stain

lactation

laparotomy

LEEP (loop electrosurgical excision procedure)

libido

LMP (last menstrual period)

lumpectomy

mastectomy

menarche

menorrhagia

menses

metrorrhagia

Monilia

morning-after pill

multipara

multiparity

nulligravida

nulliparous

oligomenorrhea

oophorectomy

ovarian follicle

PID (pelvic inflammatory disease)

preeclampsia

preterm ejaculation

salpingectomy

salpingo-oophorectomy

spermicidal

STD (sexually transmitted disease)

Trichomonas (dictated as "trich")

uterus anteverted

vasectomy

vestibulitis

wet prep

RESPIRATORY SYSTEM

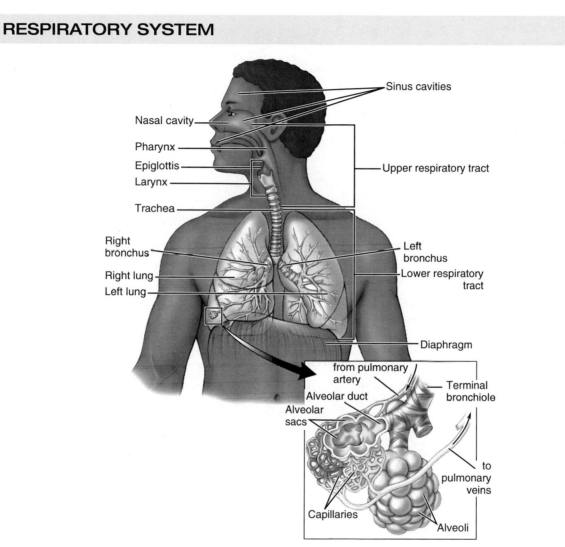

FIGURE **4-8** The respiratory system. (Modified from Brown JL: *Medical insurance made easy,* Philadelphia, 2001, WB Saunders.)

ABG (arterial blood gas)

AC (assist control—a mode for ventilator)

alveoli

AM (aerosol mask)

aortic cusp

asthma

audible

barrel chested

bedside spirometry = bedside PFT

blue bloater

bronchi

bronchial tree

bronchioles

congestion

consolidation

COPD (chronic obstructive pulmonary disease)

CPAP (continuous positive airway pressure)

CPT (chest)

crackle

croup

diffuse

D$_{LCO}$ (diffusing capacity)

dyspnea

edema

emphysema

end inspiratory/expiratory phase

ETCO monitor (end tidal CO_2 monitor)

exacerbation

exudate

FEV

fibrotic

Flo$_2$ (fractional concentration of inspired oxygen)

flow volume loop

FVC (forced vital capacity)

HHN (handheld nebulizer)

HME (2 heat and moisture 2 exchanger)

hoarse

hydration

incentive spirometer

incentive spirometry

infiltrate

infiltration

inhaler

interrogation

IPAP (inspiratory positive airway pressure)

MVV (maximum voluntary ventilator)

nebulizer

NIF (negative inspiratory force)

nocturnal

NP (nasal prongs)

NRB (nonrebreather—a mask)

O$_2$/nasal cannula

O$_2$ SAT (oxygen saturation)

partial nonbreather mask

PAT (pediatric aerosol tent)

PD (postural drainage)

PEEP (positive end-expiratory pressure)

pentamidine aerosol treatments (used to treat patients with HIV)

PF (peak flow)

PFT (pulmonary function test)

phlegm

pink puffer

pleural pH (sample of lung fluid which is used to determine pH)

pneumonia

POX (pulse oximetry)

pressure-control ventilation

PS (pressure support)

pulse oximetry

retraction

rhonchi

rhonchus

room air

RSV (respiratory syncytial virus)

SIMV (synchronized intermittent mechanical ventilation—refers to rate)

SPAG (small-particle aerosol generator)

sputum

suppurative

TC (trach collar)

USN (ultrasonic nebulizer)

VBP (vibro percussion)

VC (vital capacity)

Verazole/Ribovinin (medicine used to treat RSV)

VM (ventilation mask)

VT (tidal volume)

Normal Blood Gas Analysis

Base excess (0-1.2) mmol/L

HCO_3 (24-28) mmol/L

O_2 SAT (95-99) %

pH (7.350-7.450)

pO_2 (80-100) mmHg

pCO_2 (35-45) mmHg

Sample type—arterial

Total CO_2 (21-25) mEq/L

Draw Sites

right radial

left radial

right brachial

left brachial

right femoral

left femoral

right dorsalis pedis

left dorsalis pedis

UAC (umbilical artery catheter)

URINARY SYSTEM

24-hour urinalysis

anuria

bacteruria

benign prostatic hypertrophy

Bowman's capsule

calculi

calculus

circumcision

cystoscopy

cystourethrogram

dialysis

dribbling

dysuria

edema

efflux

Foley catheter

glomerulonephritis

GU (genitourinary)

hematuria

hesitancy

hydronephrosis

hypertension

incontinence

infection

intravenous pyelogram

lethargy

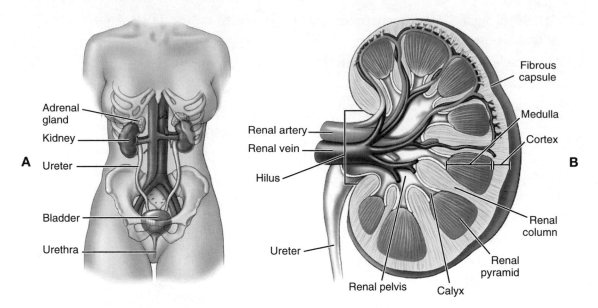

FIGURE **4-9** **A,** The urinary system. **B,** Kidney. (Modified from Brown JL: *Medical insurance made easy,* Philadelphia, 2001, WB Saunders.)

lithotripsy

micturition

nephrectomy
nephrolithiasis
nephrolithotomy
nocturia

oliguria

penile discharge
polyuria
prostatectomy
prostatitis
proteinuria
PSA
pyelonephritis

stress incontinence

UA (urinalysis)

ureteritis
ureterolithiasis
urethral discharge
urethritis
urgency
urinalysis
urine C&S
UTI (urinary tract infection)

vasectomy
voiding

Urinalysis

bilirubin
blood
color
clarity
glucose
ketones
leukocyte esterase

nitrite

pH

protein

specific gravity

urobilinogen

epithelial cells

RBCs

UA comments

WBC

Oncology

CANCER CLASSIFICATIONS

1. Do not capitalize *stage* or *grade*.
2. Use Roman numerals for cancer stages and Arabic numbers for grades.
   EXAMPLE: stage 0, stage I, stage II, stage III, stage IV; grade 1, grade 2, grade 3, grade 4.
3. CIN is an acronym for *cervical intraepithelial neoplasia*.
   EXAMPLE: CIN-1, CIN-2, CIN-3.
4. EIC is an acronym for *extensive intraductal component*.
5. Use Roman numerals to indicate Clark level, which describes invasion level of primary malignant melanoma of the skin.
   EXAMPLE: Clark level I, level II, level III, level IV.
6. Use the French-American-British Classification system (FAB) for nonlymphoid leukemia.
   EXAMPLE: M1 (no space).
7. MALT—mucosa-associated lymphoid tissue.
8. Use Roman numerals for FIGO staging of ovarian carcinoma.
   EXAMPLE: FIGO stage II.
9. TNM classification for malignant tumors.
   EXAMPLE: T_2, N_3, M_1

T	tumor size and involvement
N	regional lymph node involvement
M	extent of metastasis
T_1	2 cm or less
T_2	2-5 cm
T_3	greater than 5 cm
T_4	advanced
T_X	cannot locate
T_0	no evidence of tumor
T_{IS}	in situ

Use lowercase prefixes with TNM.

EXAMPLE: cTNM, aT$_2$

pTNM	pathology stage
oTNM	autopsy stage
yTNM	pretreatment stage
cTNM	clinical stage
stage 0	carcinoma in situ
stage I	localized carcinoma
stage II	limited to local extension
stage III	extensive
stage IV	metastasis

RADIATION ONCOLOGY TERMS

ARCTHERAPY: Rotational, moving radiation beams. The machine moves around the patient as it administers radiation.

ASYMMETRIC JAW: The area of treatment is divided into the field length (Y) and width (X). The jaw, which shapes the beam, may have two independent collimators. Asymmetric jaws are often used to prevent x-rays from diverging (like sun rays). This can be achieved by closing one independent jaw down to the central axis.

BOOST: Reduced portal implemented toward the end of the treatment course for the purpose of giving additional radiation to the original tumor site or excisional site. The boost further minimizes the dose to normal tissue.

BRACHYTHERAPY: Internal radiation, administered from an external source—a linear accelerator or cobalt machine.

CUSTOM BLOCKING: Technique using a custom-formed shield to prevent vital organs or unaffected areas close to the tumor from being irradiated.

DOSE DISTRIBUTION: Doses, represented as percentages of the total dose given, are displayed in two or three dimensions (on paper or computer) through the entire area of interest.

ELECTRONS: Ionizing particle radiation—also electrically produced.

EXTERNAL BEAM: Radiation emitted from an external source (i.e., linear accelerator or cobalt machine).

FRACTIONATION: Frequency and length of treatment course—usually once a day, 5 days/week for 2-7 weeks.

GRAY(Gy)/CENTIGRAY (cGy): A unit of radiation dose; formerly called *rad*.

INTENSITY MODULATED RADIOTHERAPY(IMRT): The latest and most promising technique in radiation therapy. Allows complete modulation of radiation dose within organs, tumors, and any area of interest. Will allow for dose escalation and tighter treatment margins, potentially affecting cure rates and recurrence rates.

ISOCENTER: The axis where all radiation beams converge. It is the point for which doses are calculated. It is also an imaginary point in space for all machine calibrations and alignments.

ISODOSE: The total dose planned to a targeted volume of tissue.

LINEAR ACCELERATOR (linac):   Machine that produces and emits high-energy radiation to kill cancer cells.

MANTLE: Type/shape of radiation portal for treating certain mediastinal tumors, such as those found in Hodgkin's lymphoma.

MEGAVOLTAGE (mV):   Radiation energy emitted from a linear accelerator—measured in millions of volts.

MONITOR UNIT (mu):   A value that is calculated and set at the linear accelerator controls to deliver a prescribed dose of radiation to a given field.

MULTILEAF COLLIMATOR (MLC):   Multiple pairs of finger-like projections built into the collimator heads of some linacs. Allows customized position for each patient so that the radiation beam can be shaped to the tumor area, blocking surrounding tissue. This takes the place of physical custom blocks.

OFF CORD: Reduced portal or additional blocking for the purpose of limiting the dose to the spinal cord. If the radiation dose exceeds the tolerance dose, the patient incurs a long-term risk of radiation myelitis, resulting in paralysis.

PARALLEL-OPPOSED: Describes portals 180 degrees apart, which treat the same volume of tissue from opposite directions.

PHOTONS: X-rays—ionizing waves electrically produced.

PORTAL: A defined area (field) of treatment. The entry/exit area of radiation beam.

RADIOTHERAPY: Radiation therapy—treatment of disease, usually malignancies, with ionizing radiation.

RESPIRATORY GATING: New technique that allows control of radiation delivery during predetermined cycles of breathing. Software directs the machine to turn the beam off when respirations move the intended target outside the preset, acceptable limits.

SIMULATION: Initial process of outlining portals, devising immobilizers, and obtaining measurements necessary for treatment planning and delivery. A special x-ray machine called a *simulator* is used for this procedure.

TELETHERAPY: Radiation therapy administered from an external source, such as a linear accelerator or cobalt machine.

WEDGED PAIR: Describes radiation portals in which accessories between beam and patient are used to evenly distribute the dose across an uneven surface. Dynamic enhanced wedges are now being used in many linacs. The dynamic wedge is a collimator jaw that sweeps across the radiation beam as treatment is being delivered.

ONCOLOGY MEDICATIONS

Achromycin

Actimmune

Actinex

actinomycin-D

Adriamycin

Adrucil

A-Hydrocort

AK-Dex

aldesleukin

Alferon N

Alkeran

allopurinol

altretamine

Amcort

Amen

A-Methapred

amethopterin

amifostine

aminoglutethimide

Ampligen

amsacrine

anabolic steroids

anagrelide

Anandron

Anapolon

anastrozole

Andro L.A.

Androcur

Androderm

androgens

Android

Andronate

Andropository

Andryl

antifungals, azole

APD

APL

Apo-Doxy

Apo-Prednisone

Apo-Tamox

Apo-Tetra

Aquest

Ara-C

Aredia

Arimidex

Aristocort

Aristocort Forte

Aristocort Intralesional

Aristospan Intra-articular

Aristospan Intralesional

Armour Thyroid

Aromasin

Articulose L.A.

Articulose-50

asparaginase

autolymphocyte therapy

Aygestin

5-AZA

bacillus Calmette-Guérin

BCNU

beta alethine

betamethasone

betamethasone acetate

betamethasone sodium phosphate

Betathine

Betnelan

Betnesol

bicalutamide

BiCNU

Biodel Implant/carmustine
bispecific antibody
Blenoxane
bleomycin sulfate
Bonefos
bromodeoxyuridine
busulfan

C.E.S.
Camptosar
carboplatin
carmustine
Casodex
CCNU
2-CdA
CeeNU
Celestone
Celestone Phosphate
Celestone Soluspan
Cenocort A-40
Cenocort Forte
Cerubidine
chimeric
chlorambucil
Chlormethine
2-chlorodeoxyadenosine
chromic phosphate
Cinolone 40
Cinonide 40
cisplatin
citrovorum factor
9-*cis* Retinoic acid
cladribine
Climara
Clinagen LA 40
colaspase
colony-stimulating factors

Colprone
Congest
Conjugated estrogens
Cortef
corticosteroids
cortisol
cortisone acetate
Cortone
Cortone Acetate
Cosmegen
coumarin
Curretab
cyclophosphamide
Cycrin
cyproterone acetate
Cytadren
cytarabine
CytoImplant
Cytomel
Cytosar
Cytosar-U
cytosine arabinoside
Cytoxan

$DAB_{389}IL-2$
dacarbazine
dactinomycin
Dalalone
Dalalone D.P.
Dalalone L.A.
daunorubicin hydrochloride
daunorubicin, liposomal
DaunoXome
2'DCF
Decadrol
Decadron
Decadron-LA

Decadron Phosphate

Deca-Durabolin

Decaject

Decaject-L.A.

Declomycin

Delatest

Delatestryl

Delestrogen

Delta-Cortef

Deltasone

demeclocycline

2'-deoxycoformycin

2'-deoxycytidine

depGynogen

depMedalone 40

depMedalone 80

Depo-Estradiol

Depofoam Encapsulated Cytarabine

DepoGen

Depoject-40

Depoject-80

Depo-Medrol

Depopred-40

Depopred-80

Depo-Predate 40

Depo-Predate 80

Depo-Provera

Depotest

Depo-Testosterone

Depo-Testosterone Cypionate

Deronil

DES-diethylstilbestrol

Dexacen LA-8

Dexacen-4

dexamethasone

dexamethasone acetate

Dexamethasone Intensol

dexamethasone sodium phosphate

dexasone

Dexasone L.A.

Dexone

Dexone 0.5

Dexone 0.75

Dexone 1.5

Dexone 4

Dexone LA

dexrazoxane

dibromodulcitol

Didronel

diethylstilbestrol diphosphate

Diflucan

Diflucan 150

5,6-dihydro-5-azacytidine

dimethyl sulfoxide

Dioval 40

Dioval XX

disaccharide

disodium clodronate

disodium clodronate tetrahydrate

docetaxel

Doryx

Doxi film

Doxil

doxorubicin

Doxy

Doxy Caps

Doxycin

doxycycline

doxycycline calcium

doxycycline hyclate

DTIC

DTIC-Dome

Durabolin

Durabolin-50

Dura-Estrin
Duragen-20
Duralone-40
Duralone-80
Dynacin

E-Cypionate
Efudex
EHDP
Eldisine
Ellence
Elliott's B solution
Elspar
Eltroxin
Emcyt
epirubicin hydrochloride
EPO
Epoetin alfa, recombinant
Epogen
Eprex
Ergamisol
Erwinase
erwinia L-asparaginase
erythropoietin, recombinant human
esterified estrogens
Estinyl
Estrace
Estraderm
estradiol
estradiol cypionate
estradiol valerate
Estragyn 5
Estragyn LA5
Estra-L 40
estramustine phosphate sodium
Estratab
Estro-A

Estro-Cyp
Estrofem
estrogens
estrogens, conjugated
estrogens, esterified
Estro-L.A.
estrone
Estrone 5
estropipate
Estro-Span
ethinyl estradiol
Ethyol
etidronate disodium
Etopophos
etoposide
etoposide phosphate
Euflex
Eulexin
Everone 200
exemestane

5-FU (fluorouracil)
Femara
Femogex
filgrastim
floxuridine
fluconazole
Fludara
fludarabine phosphate
Fluoroplex
fluorouracil
fluoxymesterone
flutamide
folinic acid
FUDR

gallium nitrate

Gamimune N

Gammagard

Gammar-IV

Ganite

gemcitabine

Gemzar

Gen-Tamoxifen

Gesterol 50

Gesterol LA 250

Gleevec

Gliadel

Gliadel Wafer

goserelin acetate

gossypol

granisetron hydrochloride

Gynogen L.A. 20

Gynogen L.A. 40

Halotestin

Hexadrol

Hexadrol Phosphate

Hexalen

hexamethylmelamine

Honvol

Human erythropoietin, recombinant

Hy/Gestrone

Hybolin Decanoate

Hybolin Improved

Hycamtin

Hydeltra T.B.A.

Hydeltrasol

Hydrea

hydrocortisone

hydrocortisone acetate

hydrocortisone cypionate

hydrocortisone sodium phosphate

hydrocortisone sodium succinate

Hydrocortone

Hydrocortone Acetate

Hydrocortone Phosphate

hydroxyprogesterone caproate

hydroxyurea

Hylutin

Idamycin

IFEX

Ifex

ImmTher

ImmuCyst

ImmuRAIT

Imuvert

interleukin-2

Intron A

iodine

Iodotope

irinotecan hydrochloride

Isovorin

itraconazole

Iveegam

IVIG

Kabolin

Kenacort

Kenacort Diacetate

Kenaject-40

Kenalog-10

Kenalog-40

Kestrone 5

ketoconazole (Nizoral)

Key-Pred 25

Key-Pred 50

Key-Pred-SP

Kidrolase

Kytril

Lanvis
letrozole
leucovorin calcium
Leukeran
Leukine
leuprolide acetate
leuprorelin
Leustatin
Leustatin injection
levamisole hydrochloride
levonorgestrel (Norplant)
Levo-T
Levothroid
levothyroxine sodium
Levoxyl
Linomide
liothyronine sodium (Cytomel)
liotrix
liposomal daunorubicin (DaunoXome)
liposome encapsulated recombinant
Liquid Pred
LL-2-1-131
lomustine
L-PAM
Lupron
Lupron Depot
Lupron Depot—3 Month
Lupron Depot—4 Month
Lupron Depot-Ped
Lysodren

Malogen in Oil
MART-1 adenoviral gene therapy
masoprocol
Matulane
mechlorethamine hydrochloride

Medralone 40
Medralone 80
medrogestone (Colprone)
Medrol
medroxyprogesterone acetate
Megace
Megace OS
megestrol
megestrol acetate
Melacine
Melimmune
melphalan
melphalan hydrochloride
Menaval-20
Menest
Meprolone
mercaptopurine
mesna
Mesnex
Metandren
methotrexate
methotrexate sodium
Methotrexate & laurocapram
Methotrexate/azone
methoxsalen
methylprednisolone
methylprednisolone acetate
methylprednisolone sodium succinate
methyltestosterone
Meticorten
miconazole (Monistat IV)
Micronor
Minocin
minocycline hydrochloride
Mithracin
mithramycin

mitomycin

mitomycin C

mitoguazone

mitolactol

mitotane

mitoxantrone

mitoxantrone hydrochloride

Monistat IV

monoclonal antibodies

Monodox

8-MOP

6-MP

Mustargen

Mutamycin

Myleran

Mymethasone

nandrolone decanoate

nandrolone phenpropionate

Natulan

Navelbine

Neo-Estrone

Neosar

Neumega rhil-11

Neupogen

NeuTrexin

Nilandron

nilutamide

Nipent

9-Nitro-20

nitrogen mustard

Nizoral

Nolvadex

Nolvadex-D

norethindrone acetate

norethisterone

norgestrel

Norlutate

Norplant

Nor-Pred T.B.A.

Nor-Q.D.

Novantrone

Novo-Doxylin

Novo-Tamoxifen

Novo-Tetra

N-trifluoroacetyl adriamycin-14-valerate

Nu-Tetra

o.p′-DDD

octreotide acetate

Ogen

Ogen 0.625

Ogen 1.25

Ogen 2.5

Oncaspar

OncoRad

Oncostate

Oncovin

ondansetron

ondansetron hydrochloride

Oradexon

Orasone 1

Orasone 5

Orasone 10

Orasone 20

Orasone 50

Oreton Methyl

Ortho-Est 0.625

Ortho-Est 1.25

OvaRex MAB-B43.13

Ovastat

Ovrette

oxaliplatin

Oxandrin

oxandrolone

Oxsoralen

Oxsoralen Lotion

Oxsoralen-Ultra

oxymetholone

oxytetracycline

oxytetracycline hydrochloride

^{32}P

PACIS

paclitaxel

pamidronate disodium

Panmycin

Panorex

Papillomavirus, human

Paraplatin

Paraplatin-AQ

Paxene

Pediapred

pegaspargase

PEG-L-asparaginase

pentostatin

Pharmorubicin PFS

Pharmorubicin RDF

phenylalanine mustard

Phosphocol P 32

Photofrin

piperazine estrone sulfate

Platinol

Platinol-AQ

plicamycin

PMS-levothyroxine sodium

PMS-progesterone

Polygam

poly-I: poly C12U

poly-ICLC

porfimer sodium

porfiromycin

Predaject-50

Predalone 50

Predalone T.B.A.

Predate 50

Predate S

Predate YBA

Predcor-25

Predcor 50

Predcor-TBA

Predicort-50

Predicort-RP

Prednicen-M

prednimustine

prednisolone

prednisolone acetate

prednisolone acetate and prednisolone

prednisolone sodium phosphate

prednisolone tebutate

prednisone

prednisone intensol

Prelone

Premarin

Premarin Intravenous

procarbazine hydrochloride

Procrit

Procytox

Prodrox

progesterone (Gesterol 50)

Proleukin

Promycin

Pro-Span

Provera

Purinethol

Rep-Pred 40

Rep-Pred 80

Retinoin

rG-CSF

rGM-CSF

rHu GM-CSF

r-HuEPO

Ricin

Ricin (Blocked) conjugated murine

r-IFN-beta

r-met HuG-CSF

Robitet

Roferon

roquinimex

Rubex

Sandoglobulin

Sandostatin

sargramostim

SD Polygam

Selestoject

Serratia marcescens extract

sodium iodine

sodium phosphate P 32

Solu-Cortef

Solu-Medrol

Solurex

Solurex LA

Sporanox

ST1-RTA

stanozolol

Sterapred

Sterapred DS

Sterecyt

stilbestrol

Stilphostrol

streptozocin

SU-101

sucralfate

Sumycin

suramin

Synthroid

T4 endonuclease V, liposome encapsulated

Tabloid

Tac-3

TA-HPV

talc, sterile aerosol

Tamofen

Tamone

Tamoplex

tamoxifen

Targretin

Taxol

Taxotere

T-Cypionate

teceleukin

Temodar

teniposide

Terramycin

Teslac

Testamone 100

Testaqua

Testex

Testoderm

Testoderm with Adhesive

testolactone

Testopel

testosterone

testosterone cypionate

testosterone enanthate

testosterone propionate

Testred

Testred Cypionate 200

Testrin-P.A.

tetracycline

tetracycline hydrochloride

tetracyclines

Tetracyn

TheraCys

thioguanine

Thioplex

thiotepa

Thyrar

Thyrogen

thyroid (Armour Thyroid, Thyrar, Thyroid
    Strong, Westhroid)

Thyroid Strong

Thyrolar

thyrotropin

Thytropar

TICE BCG

Tija

Toposar

topotecan

toremifene

Treosulfan

Tretinoin

Tretinoin LF, IV

triamcinolone

triamcinolone acetonide

triamcinolone diacetate

triamcinolone hexacetonide

Triam-Forte

Triamolone 40

Triamonide 40

Trian-A

Tri-Kort

Trilog

Trilone

trimetrexate glucuronate

Tristoject

TSH

UltraMOP

UltraMOP lotion

uracil mustard

Uromitexan

Valergen-10

Valergen-20

Valergen-40

Velban

Velbe

Venoglobulin-I

Venoglobulin-S

VePesid

Vesanoid

Vibramycin

Vibra-Tabs

vinblastine sulfate

Vincristine Sulfate

Vindesine Sulfate

Vinorelbine Tartrate

Virilon

Viron IM

Visudyne

Vivelle

VM-26

VP-16

Vumon

Vumon for Injection

Wehgen

Wellcovorin

Wellferon

Westhroid

Winpred
Winstrol

Zanosar
Zinecard

Zofran
Zoladex
Zoladex LA
Zyloprim for Injection

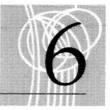

Laboratory Tests

MEDICARE CHEMISTRY PANELS

Electrolytes Panel ("Lytes")

sodium

potassium

chloride

CO_2

Hepatic Function (HFPA)

albumin

total bilirubin

direct bilirubin

alkaline phosphatase

AST

ALT

Basic Metabolic Panel (BMET)

BUN

glucose

sodium

potassium

chloride

CO_2

creatinine

Comprehensive Metabolic (CMET)

albumin

calcium

creatinine

glucose

sodium

total bilirubin

alkaline phosphatase

BUN

total protein

AST

potassium

chloride

NOTE: Basic and Comprehensive = CMET and CO_2 Hepatic and Comprehensive = CMET, DBIL, and ALT

COMPLETE BLOOD COUNT WITH DIFFERENTIAL

CBC Hemogram

WBC

RBC

HGB

HCT

MCV

MCH
MCHC
RDW
PLT
MPV

Differential

lymphocytes

neutrophils

monocytes

eosinophils

ABS neutrophils

ABS lymphocytes

ABS monocytes

ABS eosinophils

ABS basophils

platelets

RBC morphology

Rapid AMI (Acute Myocardial Infarction) Profile

troponin I

CK-MB

total CPK

CK-MB index

Urine Chemical

color

clarity

glucose

bilirubin

ketones

specific gravity

blood

pH

protein

urobilinogen

nitrate

leukocyte esterase

Microscopic Exam

RBCs—red blood cells

WBCs—white blood cells

epithelial cells

UA comments

NOTE: UA is an abbreviation for *urinalysis*. Urine type collected (i.e., catheterized, clean catch, or voided specimen). Urine hCG is a pregnancy test.

NORMAL LABORATORY VALUES

Rapid AMI Profile

troponin I	<2.6 ng/mL
CK-MB	<4.0 ng/mL
total CPK for AMI	30-135 uL
CK-MB index	<3.5

Comprehensive Metabolic

glucose	70-110 mg/dL
sodium	135-145 mEq/L
potassium	3.5-5.5 mEq/L
chloride	95-105 mEq/L
CO_2	24-30 mEq/L
anion gap	5-15 mEq/L
BUN	5-25 mg/dL
creatinine	0.5-1.4 mg/dL
calcium	8.7-10.2 mg/dL
bilirubin, total	0-1.0 mg/dL
total protein	6.3-8.2 gm/dL

albumin	3.5-5.0 gm/dL	platelets	150-400 K/uL
AST (SGOT)	8-39 U/L	MPV	7.5-10.5 fl
alkaline phosphatase	50-136 U/L		

CBC Hemogram

Differential

WBC	4.5-11.0 K/uL	lymphocytes	13-52%
RBC	4.20-5.40 M/uL	neutrophils	33-73%
hemoglobin (HGB)	12.0-16.0 gm/dL	monocytes	0-10%
hematocrit (HCT)	36.0-48.0%	eosinophils	0-4%
MCV	80.0-98.0 fl	basophils	0-2%
MCH	27.0-32.0 pg	ABS neutrophils	1.8-7.7 K/uL
MCHC	32.0-36.0 gm/dL	ABS lymphocytes	1.0-4.8 K/uL
RDW	11.5-14.5%	ABS monocytes	0-0.8 K/uL
		ABS basophils	0-0.2 K/uL

LABORATORY TESTS

NOTE: If you were transcribing the actual test, you would capitalize the test. However, in general transcription, you would not capitalize the test unless it was a proper name.

24-hour urine
3-hour glucose tolerance test
5-hour glucose tolerance test
ABO RH blood group & type
Accutane panel
acetylcholine receptor antibody
acetylcholinesterase
acid-fast smear
acid phosphatase, enzymatic
acute myocardial infarction profile
adrenocorticotropic hormone
AFP material (serum)
albumin
alcohol (blood ETOH)
aldolase
aldosterone
alkaline phosphatase
alpha fetoprotein
alprazolam

ALT
aluminum
amended metabolic panel
amenorrhea profile
amikacin
amitriptyline
ammonia
amoeba
amoxapine
amphetamine confirmation
amylase
anemia profile
angiotensin-1-converting enzyme
anticentromere
antidiuretic hormone
anti-DNA
anti-DNA B titer
antimitochondrial antibody
antineutrophil cytoplasm AB

antinuclear antibody (ANA)

antiparietal cell antibody

antiskin antibody

anti–smooth muscle antibody

antithrombin III

antithyroid AB

arthritis profile

ASO titer

AST (SGOT)

atypical pneumonia antibody

Aventyl (nortriptyline)

bacterial antigen panel

barbiturate confirmation

basic metabolic panel (BMET)

benzodiazepine confirmation

beta 2 microglobulin

bilirubin

bilirubin, direct neonatal

bilirubin, neonatal

bleeding time

blood exposure panel

blood smear review

bone marrow

Bordetella pertussis smear

Brucella antibody screen

BUN (blood urea nitrogen)

CO_2 content (bicarbonate)

CA27.29

calcium

calcium ionized

cancer antigen 125

cancer antigen T 15-3

Candida antibody screen

carbamazepine

carbohydrate antigen 19-9

carboxyhemoglobin (Carb. Monox.)

cardiolipin antibody

carotene

catecholamines, plasma fraction

CBC with diff

CD4 count

ceruloplasmin

Chlamydia antigen DFA smear

chloride

cholesterol

Chlamydia antibody titer (IFA)

Chlamydia pneumonia antibody

Chlamydia/GC DNA-probe

CK-MB

clonazepam

Clostridium difficile (stool)

cocaine metabolite

Coccidioides antibody screen

comprehensive O&P (feces)

complement, total hemolytic

complete blood count (CBC)

comprehensive metabolic panel

cord blood, BB

cortisol, serum

cortisol, urine free

CPK

C-reactive protein, quant.

crossmatch (transfuse PRC), BB

cryoglobulin screen

cryoprecipitate—transfuse, BB

cryptococcal antigen titer

Cryptosporidium AG test (feces)

CSF (cell count cerebrospinal fluid)

CSF protein

CSF spinal fluid

CSF, VDRL (spinal fluid)

culture, aerobic

culture, AFB

culture, anaerobic

culture, blood, fungus

culture, Bordetella pertussis

culture, breast milk

culture, catheter tip

culture, Chlamydia

culture, CSF (cerebrospinal fluid)

culture, cytomegalovirus—urine

culture, ear—not ear fluid

culture, eye—not eye fluid

culture, fungal—not CSF

culture, fungus CSF

culture, group B strep

culture, herpes

culture, Legionella

culture, nasopharyngeal

culture, respiratory

culture, routine

culture, skin fungus

culture, stool

culture, throat beta strep GP A

culture, urine

culture, viral

cytomegalovirus AB (IGG/IGM)

D-dimer

dehydroepiandrosterone sulfate

Depakene (valproic acid)

Dilantin (phenytoin)

direct Coombs' antiglobulin, BB

drug abuse profile (urine)

electrolytes panel

ENA screen profile (Sjögren's)

Epstein-Barr virus—AB titer

Epstein-Barr virus—early

Epstein-Barr virus—nuclear

erythropoietin

eosinophil smear, nonblood

estradiol

factor 8 transfusion, BB

factor 9 transfusion, BB

factor IX activity

factor V mutation

factor VIII (8) comp. profile

factor VIII activity

febrile agglutinins

feces, fat undigested

feces, Giardia antigen test

feces, occult blood

feces, pH

feces, reducing substances

feces, rotavirus antigen test

feces, WBC smear

ferritin

fetal fibronectin

fetal hemoglobin

fetal maturity panel

FFP (fresh frozen plasma), BB

fibrinogen

fluid, pH

fluid, specific gravity

FNA cytology

folate, RBC

folate, serum

follicle-stimulating hormone

free PSA ratio

free T_4

FTA-ABS IgM

FTA-ABS serology

fungal antibody screen

G6PD screen

gabapentin

galactose I phosphate, uridyl

gastric occult blood

gastrin

GC DNA-probe

GC screen—get culture media

gentamicin/Garamycin—post

gentamicin/Garamycin—PRE

GGTP

Giardia/Crpto O&P (feces)

glomerular basement membrane AB

glucose

glucose (serum)

glucose (bedside—Accu-Chek)

glycosylated hemoglobin (A_{1C})

Gram stain

GTT OB screen

GYN cytology

H&H (hemoglobin/hematocrit)

haptoglobin

hCG, serum (pregnancy test)

Heinz body screen

hemochromatosis genetic
    screen

hepatic function panel

hepatitis A IgM antibody

hepatitis B surface antigen

hepatitis C (HCV)

hepatitis profile

herpes simplex I virus antibody

herpes simplex II virus antibody

herpes virus antigen DFA smear

HGB electrophoresis

Histoplasma antibody

HIV antibody screen

HIV P-24

HIVC

homocysteine

human growth hormone

immunofixation, serum

immunoglobulin A, D, E, G, M

immunoglobulin (IgA, IgG, IgM)

India ink prep

indirect Coombs'

inhibitor study (Protime Inhib)

inpatient surgical

insulin antibody

insulin level

iron

iron profile

Kleihauer Betke (fetal) stain, BB

Klonopin

KOH prep (fungal preparation)

lactic acid

latex allergy test

LDH

lead, serum

Legionella pneumonia antibody

Legionella pneumonia urinary AG

leptospirosis AB

leukocyte esterase stain

leukocyte peroxidase stain

LFP chemistry panel

lipase

lipid profile

lipoprotein electrophoresis

lithium

lupus anticoagulant profile

luteinizing hormone

lyme disease AB titer

magnesium

malaria screen

marijuana metabolite

menopausal profile

metabolic screen

methemoglobin

microalbumin/creatinine ratio

misc. battery 1, 3, 4, 5

mono test

mumps antibody

mycoplasma antibody (IgG & IgM)

myoglobin, serum

mysoline

nongyn cytology

oligoclonal banding CSF

opiate confirmation

osmolality, serum

Osteomark (NTX-Telopeptide)

pancreatic islet cell antibody

parathyroid hormone C terminal

parathyroid hormone N terminal

paratyphoid A

paratyphoid B

parvovirus B19

PAS stain

PCP

PCP confirmation

phenobarbital

pH

PKU (phenylketonuria)

platelet AB drug dependent

platelet AB heparin dependent

platelet aggregation profile

platelet antibody ID

platelet antibody screen

platelet count

platelet transfusion, BB

potassium, serum

prealbumin

procainamide &/or

prolactin

prostate profile

prostate-specific antigen (PSA)

protein C panel

protein C&S panel

protein S panel

proteus

proteus OX2

proteus OXK

PSA screen

PT (Protime)

PTH intact

PTT (partial thromboplastin time)

quinidine

rapid influenza

RAST (Pollen Profile Allergy Test)

RBC antibody titer, BB

renal panel

renin

respiratory syncytial antigen

reticulocyte count (RETIC)

RH type-RH(D) type, BB

rheumatoid factor (RA TEST)

Rhogam (RH IB) transfusion, BB

Rhogam (RH IG PP/2ND TRIM.), BB

Rocky Mt. spotted fever titer

RPR (rapid plasma reagin)

rubella AB—quant (IgG & IgM)

rubella AB immune status

rubella antibody

salicylate (aspirin)

Schilling's phase 1, 2

sed rate (Westergren ESR)

semen analysis (fertility)

semen analysis (postvasectomy)

serum creatinine

serum protein electrophoresis

sickle cell screen

Sinequan

sodium

stone analysis

strep A screen

sweat chloride/cystic fibrosis

synovial/joint fluid cnt

T_3 free

T_3, total (T_3 by RIA)

T_4

THC confirmation

theophylline (aminophylline)

therapeutic phlebotomy, BB

thrombin time

thyroid-binding globulin

thyroid profile

thyroid profile B

thyroid-stimulating hormone

tick exam

T-lymph panel (cell immune)

tobramycin, post (peak)

tobramycin, pre

topiramate

torch screen

total iron-binding capacity

total protein

Toxoplasma antibody

transferrin

transfusion reaction, BB

trazodone

triglyceride

troponin I

type & hold (type & screen), BB

typhoid H

typhoid O

uric acid, serum

urinalysis

urine (24-hour)

urine creatinine clearance

urine drug screen

urine free hydroxyproline

urine glucose

urine microscopic add

urine microscopic only

urine osmolality

urine potassium

urine protein electrophoresis

urine without microscopic

urine, 12-hour urea nitrogen

urine, 24-hour calcium

urine, 24-hour catecholamines

urine, 24-hour metanephrine

urine, 24-hour oxalate

urine, 24-hour porphobilinogen

urine, 24-hour protein

urine, 24 VMA

urine, marijuana (cannabinoids)

urine, microalbumin

urine, opiates

urine, random total protein

urine, reducing substance

urine, sodium

urine, sodium 24-hour

urine, specific gravity

vaginal pathogens SCRN by DNA

vancomycin, post, peak

vancomycin, pre (trough)

varicella AB (chicken pox) titer

varicella (chicken pox) immune

vasoactive intest. polypeptide

vitamin B_1

vitamin B_{12}

vitamin B_{12} & folate

vitamin E

von Willebrand (ristocetin)

WBC (white blood cell count)

wet prep, vaginal smear

Xylocaine

xylose

Zarontin

LABORATORY TEST ABBREVIATIONS

ABO (blood type)

ABO/Rh (blood type/blood group)

Acetaminophen (Tylenol)

acetone

acid-fast bacillus stains

acid phosphatase

aerobic culture

AFB stains

Alb, serum/plasma (Alb)

alanine aminotransferase (ALT/SGPT)

albumin, serum/plasma (Alb)

alkaline phosphatase (ALP)

ALP (alkaline phosphatase)

ALT (alanine aminotransferase)

ammonia

amylase, body fluid

amylase, serum/plasma

amylase, urine

anaerobic culture

antibody elution (eluate)

antibody identification (antibody panel, antibody titer)

antibody panel (antibody titer, antibody ID)

antibody screen (indirect antiglobulin test)

antibody titer (titer)

aspartate aminotransferase (AST/SGOT)

aspirin (salicylate)

AST (aspartate aminotransferase/SGOT)

bedside glucose (GLUBS)

bilirubin, direct

bilirubin, direct, diazo, neonatal

bilirubin, direct, spectrophotometric, neonatal

bilirubin, total

bilirubin, urine, manual (Ictotest)

biopsy, liver

biopsy, skin

bleeding time (BT/Surgicutt)

blood culture

blood group, ABO (ABO, blood type)

blood group, Rh (Rh, blood type)

blood, stool (guaiac, stool blood)

blood type/blood group (ABO/Rh)

blood type & screen, hold (type, screen & hold)

body fluid analysis

bone marrow (assistance and preparation of smears)

BUN, serum (blood urea nitrogen, urea)

calcium, serum/plasma (CA)

CBC with differential (CBCD, complete blood count with differential)

CBC without differential (CBC, hemogram)

chloride, serum/plasma (Cl)

cholesterol

cholesterol, HDL (high-density lipoprotein)

CK (creatine kinase, CPK)

CK-MB

Clinitest, urine (manual reducing substances, urine)

CMV (cytomegalovirus culture)

compatibility test (crossmatch)

complete blood count w/ differential (CBCD)

complete blood count without differential (CBC, hemogram)

Coombs' test, direct (direct Coombs', direct screen, DAT)

Coombs' test, indirect (indirect Coombs', indirect screen)

cord blood battery (cord blood workup)

cord blood workup

CPK (CK, creatine kinase)

CO_2, serum

creatine kinase (CK)

creatinine, serum/plasma

creatinine, urine

crossmatch (compatibility test)

cryptococcal antigen testing

crystal ID, fluid

CSF analysis (spinal fluid analysis)

culture, aerobic

culture, anaerobic

culture, blood

culture, cytomegalovirus (CMV)

culture, fungus (fungus culture)

culture, respiratory

culture, spinal fluid

culture, stool

culture, throat

culture, urine

cytology, gynecologic (Pap smear)

cytomegalovirus culture (CMV)

DAT (Coombs' test direct/direct Coombs')

D-dimer, semiquantitative

eluate (antibody elution)

enteric pathogens (stool culture)

eosinophil, urine (eos, urine)

ESR (erythrocyte sedimentation rate, sed rate)

erythrocyte sedimentation rate (ESR, sed rate)

fat, urine

fat, quantitative, stool (fecal)

Fe (iron)

fecal fat, qualitative

fecal fat, quantitative

fetal cell stain (Kleihauer Betke stain)

fibrinogen

fine needle aspirations

flu test (influenza testing)

free T_4 (free thyroxine, fT_4, T_4f)

fungus culture (culture, fungus)

gamma glutamyl transferase (GGT)

GGT (gamma glutamyl transferase)

GLUBS (bedside glucose)

glucose, bedside (GLUBS)

glucose, body fluid

glucose, CSF

glucose, serum/plasma

glucose, urine, quantitative

Gram stain

group A strep screen

group B beta strep screen

guaiac (occult blood, stool blood)

gynecologic cytology (Pap smear)

H & H (hemoglobin/hematocrit)

hCG quantitative, serum

hCG, urine, quantitative (human chorionic gonadotropin, urine quantitative)

HDL cholesterol (high-density lipoprotein)

hemoglobin/hematocrit (H & H)

hemogram (complete blood count w/o differential)

herpes

high-density lipoprotein (HDL)

human chorionic gonadotropin, quantitative, serum (hCG, quan. serum)

human chorionic gonadotropin, urine quantitative (hCG quan. urine)

Ictotest, urine (manual bilirubin, urine/ Ictotest)

India ink prep

indirect antiglobulin test (antibody screen)

indirect Coombs' test (Indirect screen, Coombs' test indirect)

infectious mononucleosis test (monotest)

influenza testing (flu test)

intravenous RhoGAM (Win Rho)

iron (Fe)

iron-binding capacity (TIBC)

ketones, serum

K (potassium)

Kleihauer Betke stain (fetal cell stain)

KOH prep

lactic acid, CSF

lactic dehydrogenase (LD)

LAP stain (leukocyte alkaline phosphatase stain)

LD serum (LDH, lactic dehydrogenase)

LDH, body fluid

LDH, serum (LD/lactic dehydrogenase)

leukocyte alkaline phosphatase stain (LAP stain)

lipase

lithium (Li)

liver biopsy (Bx, liver)

magnesium, serum/plasma

malaria screening

Mg, serum/plasma (magnesium)

microalbumin, semiquantitative, urine

mono (infectious mononucleosis test, monotest)

mononucleosis test (mono, monotest, infectious mononucleosis test)

monotest (infectious mononucleosis test)

nongynecologic brushings

nongynecologic fluid specimens

nongynecologic smears

nongynecologic smears for Pneumocystis or fungal stain

nonspecific esterase stain (NSE stain)

NSE stain (nonspecific esterase stain)

occult blood (guaiac, stool blood)

Pap smear (gynecologic cytology)

partial thromboplastin time (PTT)

PAS (periodic acid-Schiff) stain

periodic acid-Schiff stain (PAS stain)

perox stain (peroxidase stain)

peroxidase stain (perox stain)

pH, stool (fecal pH, stool for pH)

phenytoin

phlebotomy (therapeutic phlebotomy)

phosphorus, serum/plasma (PO_4)

PLT automated (platelet count only, automated)

PO_4, serum/plasma (PO_4, phosphorus)

POC (products of conception)

polys in stool (WBCs in stool, smear for WBCs)

postpartum workup (RhoGAM workup, RhIG)

potassium, serum/plasma (K)

pregnancy test, quan (see hCG or human chorionic gonadotropin, quan.)

pregnancy test, qual. (see hCG or human chorionic gonadotrophin, qual.)

prenatal Screen I (prenatal workup)

prenatal Screen II (prenatal workup)

prenatal workup (prenatal screen)

products of conception (POC)

protein, total, CSF

protein, total, serum/plasma

protein, total, urine

protime (PT, prothrombin time)

prothrombin time (PT/protime)

PT (Protime/prothrombin time)

PTI (Protime mixing study)

PTT (Partial thromboplastin time)

PTTI (PTT mixing study)

rapid plasma reagin

reducing substances

respiratory culture

Rh (blood group)

RhIG, postpartum (RhoGAM workup)

RhoGAM, intravenous (Win Rho)

RhoGAM workup (RhIG, postpartum workup)

routine urinalysis (UA)

RPR (rapid plasma reagin)

salicylate

sed rate (sedimentation rate, ESR, erythrocyte sedimentation rate)

sedimentation rate (ESR, erythrocyte sedimentation rate, sed rate)

semen analysis

sensitivity

SGPT (alanine aminotransferase; ALT)

Sickledex (sickle cell screen)

skin biopsy (Bx, skin)

smear for WBCs (WBCs in stool, polys in stool)

sodium, serum/plasma (Na)

sodium, urine (Na, urine)

spinal fluid analysis (CSF analysis)

spinal fluid culture

strep screen (group A strep)

strep screen (group B beta strep screen)

stool blood (guaiac, occult blood)

stool culture

stool fat (fecal fat)

stool pH (fecal pH)

T_3 uptake (T_3/triiodothyronine)

T_4 free (free thyroxine, fT_4, T_4f)

T_4 total (T_4, thyroxine total)

therapeutic phlebotomy (phlebotomy)

throat culture

thyroid profile (includes T_4, T_3 uptake, FTI)

thyroid-stimulating hormone (TSH)

thyroxine free (T_4f, fT_4)

TIBC (total iron-binding capacity)

tissue specimen

triglycerides

troponin-I

TSH (thyroid-stimulating hormone)

type, screen & hold (blood type & screen)

UA (routine urinalysis)

urea, serum (BUN/blood urea nitrogen)

uric acid, serum

urinalysis, routine

urine culture

valproic acid

vancomycin

WBC automated (WBC only, automated)

WBCs in stool (smear for WBCs, polys in stool)

WBC only, automated (white blood cell count, automated)

wet prep

white blood cell count only, automated (WBC)

Win Rho (intravenous RhoGAM)

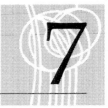

Microbiology

GRAM-POSITIVE AEROBIC BACTERIA

Micrococcaceae

ABBREVIATION	ORGANISM	SYNONYM/OTHER DESIGNATION
L. monocytogenes	Listeria monocytogenes	
Micrococcus sp.	Micrococcus species	M. aglis
		M. kristinae
		M. luteus
		M. lylae
		M. nishinomiyaensis
		M. roseus
		M. sedentarius
		M. varlans
S. arlettae	Staphylococcus arlettae	
S. aureus	Staphylococcus aureus	
S. auricularis	Staphylococcus auricularis	
S. capitis	Staphylococcus capitis	
S. carnosus	Staphylococcus carnosus	
S. cohnii	Staphylococcus cohnii	
S. epidermidis	Staphylococcus epidermidis	
S. equorum	Staphylococcus equorum	
S. gallinarum	Staphylococcus gallinarum	
S. haemolyticus	Staphylococcus haemolyticus	
S. hominis	Staphylococcus hominis	
S. hyicus hyicus	Staphylococcus hyicus, subsp. hyicus	
S. intermedius	Staphylococcus intermedius	
S. kloosii	Staphylococcus kloosii	

ABBREVIATION	ORGANISM	SYNONYM/OTHER DESIGNATION
S. lentus	Staphylococcus lentus	
S. lugdunensis	Staphylococcus lugdunensis	
S. saprophyticus	Staphylococcus saprophyticus	
S. sciuri	Staphylococcus sciuri	
S. simulans	Staphylococcus simulans	
S. warneri	Staphylococcus warneri	
S. xylosus	Staphylococcus xylosus	

Streptococcaceae

ABBREVIATION	ORGANISM	SYNONYM/OTHER DESIGNATION
Aero. viridans	Aerococcus viridans	
Ec. avium	Enterococcus avium	Group D enterococcus: St. avium
Ec. durans	Enterococcus durans	Group D enterococcus: St. durans
Ec. faecalis	Enterococcus faecalis	Group D enterococcus: St. faecalis
Ec. faecium	Enterococcus faecium	Group D enterococcus: St. faecium
G. morbillorum	Gemella morbillorum	Streptococcus morbillorum group B
St. agalactiae H	Streptococcus agalactiae Beta-hemolytic	Group B
St. agalact non-H	Streptococcus agalactiae nonhemolytic	Group B
St. angin/milleri	Streptococcus anginosus/ Streptococcus milleri	
St. bovis I	Streptococcus bovis I	Group D, nonenterococcus
St. bovis II	Streptococcus bovis II	Group D, nonenterococcus
St. const/milleri	Streptococcus constellatus/ Streptococcus milleri	
St. equi/equisim	Streptococcus equi/ Streptococcus equisimilis	Group C
St. equinus	Streptococcus equinus	Group D, nonenterococcus
St. equinus II	Streptococcus equinus (mannose positive, arabinose negative)	Group D, nonenterococcus
St. inter/milleri	Streptococcus intermedius/ Streptococcus milleri	St. intermedius
St. mitis	Streptococcus mitis	Viridans streptococcus

ABBREVIATION	ORGANISM	SYNONYM/OTHER DESIGNATION
St. mitis II	Streptococcus mitis (arginine positive)	Viridans streptococcus: St. mitior
St. mutans	Streptococcus mutans	Viridans streptococcus
St. pneumoniae	Streptococcus pneumoniae	Pneumococcus
St. pyogenes	Streptococcus pyogenes	Group A
St. salivarius	Streptococcus salivarius	Viridans streptococcus
St. sanguis I	Streptococcus sanguis I	Viridans streptococcus
St. sanguis II	Streptococcus sanguis II	Viridans streptococcus: dextran-positive St. mitior
St. zooepidemicus	Streptococcus zooepidemicus	Group C

GRAM-NEGATIVE AEROBIC BACTERIA

Gram-Negative Glucose Fermenters

ABBREVIATION	ORGANISM	SYNONYM/OTHER DESIGNATION
Aer. hydro group	Aeromonas hydrophila group	Aeromonas caviae Aeromonas hydrophila Aeromonas veronii
Ced. davisae	Cedecea davisae	Enteric group 15
Ced. lapegei	Cedecea lapegei	Enteric group 15
Ced. neteri	Cedecea neteri	Enteric group 15
Cedecea sp. 3	Cedecea species 3	
Cedecea sp. 5	Cedecea species 5	
Chrom. violaceum	Chromobacterium violaceum	
Chr. indologenes	Chryseobacterium indologenes	Flavobacterium indologenes
Chr. meningo	Chryseobacterium meningosepticum	Flavobacterium meningosepticum
Cit. amalonaticus	Citrobacter amalonaticus	Levinea amalonaticus
Cit. freundii	Citrobacter freundii	
Cit. koseri	Citrobacter koseri	Citrobacter diversus
Ed. tarda	Edwardsiella tarda	
Ent. aerogenes	Enterobacter aerogenes	
Ent. agglomerans	Enterobacter agglomerans	
Ent. amnigenus 1	Enterobacter amnigenus 1	
Ent. amnigenus 2	Enterobacter amnigenus 2	
Ent. asburiae	Enterobacter asburiae	Enteric group 17
Ent. cloacae	Enterobacter cloacae	

ABBREVIATION	ORGANISM	SYNONYM/OTHER DESIGNATION
Ent. gergoviae	Enterobacter gergoviae	
Ent. intermedium	Enterobacter intermedium	
Ent. sakazakii	Enterobacter sakazakii	Enterobacter cloacae, yellow pigmented
Ent. taylorae	Enterobacter taylorae	Enteric group 19
E. coli	Escherichia coli	
E. fergusonii	Escherichia fergusonii	Enteric group 10
E. hermannii	Escherichia hermannii	Enteric group 11
E. vulneris	Escherichia vulneris	Enteric group 1, Alma I
Ewin. americana	Ewingella americana	
Haf. alvei	Hafnia alvei	Enterobacter Hafnia
Kl. ornithinolytt	Klebsiella ornithinolytica	Enteric group 47
Kl. oxytoca	Klebsiella oxytoca	
Kl. ozaenae	Klebsiella ozaenae	
Kl. pneumoniae	Klebsiella pneumoniae	
Kl. rhinoscler	Klebsiella rhinoscleromatis	
Klu. ascorbata	Kluyvera ascorbata	Enteric group 8
Klu. cryocrescens	Kluyvera cryocrescens	Enteric group 8
Lec. adecarboxy	Leclercia adecarboxylata	Enteric group 41
Leminorella sp.	Leminorella species	Enteric group 57
M. wisconsensis	Moellerella wisconsensis	Enteric group 46
Morg. morganii	Morganella morganii	Proteus morganii
Past. aerogenes	Pasteurella aerogenes	
Past. multocida	Pasteurella multocida	
Past-Actin sp.	Pasteurella-Actinobacillus species	
Pl. shigelloides	Plesiomonas shigelloides	Aeromonas shigelloides
Prt. mirabilis	Proteus mirabilis	
Prt. penneri	Proteus penneri	Proteus vulgaris biogroup 1
Prt. vulgaris	Proteus vulgaris	
Prv. alcal 1-2	Providencia alcalifaciens 1-2	
Prv. rettgeri	Providencia rettgeri	Proteus rettgeri biogroups 1-4
Prv. rustigianii	Providencia rustigianii	Providencia alcalifaciens biogroup 3
Prv. stuartii	Providencia stuartii	
Prv. stuartii Urea (+)	Providencia stuartii Urea (+)	Proteus rettgen biogroup 5
Sal. choleraesuis	Salmonella choleraesuis	

ABBREVIATION	ORGANISM	SYNONYM/OTHER DESIGNATION
Sal. paratyphi A	Salmonella paratyphi A	
Sal. typhi	Salmonella typhi	
Sal/Arizona	Salmonella/Arizona	Arizona hinshawii
Salmonella sp.	Salmonella species	Salmonella enteritidis
Ser. fonticola	Serratia fonticola	Serratia fonticola
Ser. liquefaciens	Serratia liquefaciens	
Ser. marcescens	Serratia marcescens	
Ser. odorifera 1	Serratia odorifera I	
Ser. odorifera 2	Serratia odorifera 2	
Ser. plymuthica	Serratia plymuthica	
Ser. rubidaea	Serratia rubidaea	
Sh. sonnei	Shigella sonnei	Shigella group D
Shigella sp.	Shigella species	Shigella groups C, A, and B
	Shigella boydii	
	Shigella dysenteriae	
	Shigella flexneri	
Tatum. ptyseos	Tatumella ptyseos	
Vib. alginolyt	Vibrio alginolyticus	
Vib. cholerae	Vibrio cholerae	
Vib. damsela	Vibrio damsela	
Vlb. fluvialis	Vibrio fluvialis	CDC group EF-6; group F Vibrio
Vib. hollisae	Vibrio hollisae	CDC group EF-13
Vib. mimicus	Vibrio mimicus	Vibrio cholera, sucrose (–)
Vib. parahaemolyt	Vibrio parahaemolyticus	
Vib. vulnificus	Vibrio vulnificus	Lactose (+) halophilic Vibrio
Y. entero group	Yersinia enterocolitica group	Yersinia enterocolitica
		Yersinia frederiksenii
		Yersinia intermedia
		Yersinia kristensenii
Y. pestis	Yersinia pestis	
Y. pseudotb	Yersinia pseudotuberculosis	
Y. ruckeri	Yersinia ruckeri	Red mouth bacterium
Yok. regensburgei	Yokenella regensburgei	Koserella trabulsii

Gram-Negative Glucose Nonfermenters and Slow Glucose Fermenters

ABBREVIATION	ORGANISM	SYNONYM/OTHER DESIGNATION
Ac. baum/haem	Acinetobacter baumannii/ Acinetobacter haemolyticus	Acinetobacter anitratus/haemolyticus
Ac. iwoffli	Acinetobacter iwoffli	Genospecies 8 and 9
Ag. radiobacter	Agrobacterium radiobacter	
Al. xylosoxidans	Alcaligenes xylosoxidans, subsp. xylosoxidans	Alcaligenes xylosoxidans
Alcaligenes sp.	Alcaligenes species	Alcaligenes denitrificans
	Alcaligenes xylosoxidans, subsp. denitrificans	
	Alcaligenes faecalis	
	Alcaligenes odorans	
Brg. zoohelcum	Bergeyella zoohelcum	Weeksella zoohelcum
B. bronchiseptica	Bordetella bronchiseptica	Bordetella bronchicanis
Brk. cepacia	Burkholderia cepacia	Pseudomonas cepacia
Brk. pickettii	Burkholderia pickettii	Pseudomonas pickettii
Brk. pseudomallei	Burkholderia pseudomallei	Pseudomonas pseudomallei
CDC IV C-2	CDC IV C-2	
Chr. indologenes	Chryseobacterium indologenes	Flavobacterium indologenes
Chr. meningo (NF)	Chryseobacterium meningosepticum	Flavobacterium meningosepticum
Cry. luteola	Chryseomonas luteola	CDC group VE-1
Com. acidovorans	Comamonas acidovorans	Pseudomonas acidovorans
Emp. brevis	Empedobacter brevis	Flavobacterium breve
Flv. oryzihabitans	Flavimonas oryzihabitans	CDC group VE-2
Fl. odoratum	Flavobacterium odoratum	CDC M IV F
Moraxella sp.	Moraxella species	Moraxella atlantae
		Moraxella lacunata
		Moraxella non-liquefaciens
		Moraxella osloensis
		Moraxella phenylpyruvica
		Oligella urethralis
Och. anthropi	Ochrobactrum anthropi	Achromobacter sp. VD-1,2
Olg. ureolytica	Oligella ureolytica	CDC group IV E
Past. multo SF	Pasteurella multocida	
Past-Actin sp. SF	Pasteurella-Actinobacillus species	

ABBREVIATION	ORGANISM	SYNONYM/OTHER DESIGNATION
Ps. aeruginosa	Pseudomonas aeruginosa	
Ps. fluor/putida	Pseudomonas fluorescens/ Pseudomonas putida	
Ps. stutzeri	Pseudomonas stutzeri	CDC group VB
Pseudomonas sp.	Pseudomonas species	
	Brevundimonas diminuta	
	Brevundimonas vesicularis	
	Pseudomonas alcaligenes	
	Pseudomonas pseudoalcaligenes	
Sh. putrefaciens	Shewanella putrefaciens	Pseudomonas putrefaciens
Sph. multivorum	Sphingobacterium multivorum	Flavobacterium multivorum
Sph. spiritivorum	Sphingobacterium spiritivorum	Flavobacterium spiritivorum
Sp. paucimobilis	Sphingomonas paucimobilis	Pseudomonas paucimobilis
Stn. maltophilia	Stenotrophomonas maltophilia	Xanthomonas maltophilia
Vibrio sp. SF	Vibrio species	
	Vibrio alginolyticus	
	Vibrio damsela	
	Vibrio fluvialis	
	Vibrio hollisae	
	Vibrio parahaemolyticus	
	Vibrio vulnificus	
Wk. virosa	Weeksella virosa	CDC group II F
Y. pseudotb. SF	Yersinia pseudotuberculosis	

YEAST AND YEAST-LIKE MICROORGANISMS

ABBREVIATION	ORGANISM	SYNONYM/OTHER DESIGNATION
B. capitatus	Blastoschizomyces capitatus	Trichosporon capitatum Geotrichum capitatum
C. albicans	Candida albicans	
C. catenulata	Candida catenulata	Candida ravautii
C. guilliermondii	Candida guilliermondii	Pichia guilliermondii (perfect state)
C. humicola	Candida humicola	
C. krusei	Candida krusei	Isaatchenkia orientalis (perfect state)
C. lambica	Candida lambica	

ABBREVIATION	ORGANISM	SYNONYM/OTHER DESIGNATION
C. lipolytica	Candida lipolytica	Saccharomycopsis lipolytica (perfect state)
C. lusitaniae	Candida lusitaniae	Clavispora lusitaniae (perfect state)
C. parapsilosis	Candida parapsilosis	
C. pseudotropical	Candida pseudotropicalis	Candida kefyr
		Candida macedoniensis
		Kluyvermyces marxianus (perfect state)
C. rugosa	Candida rugosa	
C. stellatoidea	Candida stellatoidea	
C. tropicalis	Candida tropicalis	
C. tropicalis (sn)	Candida tropicalis	Candida paratropicalis (sucrose negative)
C. viswanathii	Candida viswanathii	
C. zeylanoides	Candida zeylanoides	
Cr. albidus	Cryptococcus albidus	Cryptococcus albidus var albidus
		Cryptococcus albidus var diffluens
Cr. ater	Cryptococcus ater	
Cr. gastricus	Cryptococcus gastricus	
Cr. laurentii	Cryptococcus laurentii	
Cr. melibiosum	Cryptococcus melibiosum	
Cr. neoformans	Cryptococcus neoformans	Filobasidiella neoformans (perfect state)
Cr. terreus	Cryptococcus terreus	Cryptococcus himalayensis
Cr. uniguttulatus	Cryptococcus uniguttulatus	
Geotrichum sp.	Geotrichum species	
H. anomala	Hansenula anomala	Candida pelliculosa (imperfect state)
H. polymorpha	Hansenula polymorpha	Hansenula angusta
K. lactis	Kluyveromyces lactis	Kluyveromyces marxianus var. lactis
		Candida sphaerica (imperfect state)
P. farinosa	Pichia farinosa	
Pr. wickerhamii	Prototheca wickerhamii	
Prototheca sp.	Prototheca species	Prototheca zopfii

ABBREVIATION	ORGANISM	SYNONYM/OTHER DESIGNATION
		Prototheca moriformis
		Prototheca stagnora
R. glutinis	Rhodotorula glutinis	Rhodosporidium sp. (perfect state)
R. minuta	Rhodotorula minuta	
R. rubra	Rhodotorula rubra	Rhodotorula pilimaniae
S. cerevisiae	Saccharomyces cerevisiae	Saccharomyces uvarum
Sp. salmonicolor	Sporobolomyces salmonicolor	Sporidobolus samonicolor (perfect state)
T. candida	Torulopsis candida	Candida famata
		Debaryomyces hansenii (perfect state)
T. glabrata	Torulopsis glabrata	Candida glabrata
T. inconspicua	Torulopsis inconspicua	Candida inconspicua
T. pintolopesii	Torulopsis pintolopesii	Candida pintolopesii;
		Saccharomyces telluris (perfect state)
Tr. beigelii	Trichosporon beigelii	Trichosporon cutaneum

ANAEROBES

Anaerobic Cocci

ABBREVIATION	ORGANISM	SYNONYM/OTHER DESIGNATION
Acida. fermentans	Acidaminococcus fermentans	
Ps. anaerobius	Peptostreptococcus anaerobius	
Ps. asaccharolyt	Peptostreptococcus asaccharolyticus	Peptococcus asaccharolyticus
Ps. magnus	Peptostreptococcus magnus	Peptococcus magnus
Ps. prevotii	Peptostreptococcus prevotii	Peptococcus prevotii
Ps. tetradius	Peptostreptococcus tetradius	Gaffkya anaerobia
S. sacchrolyt	Staphylococcus saccharolyticus	Peptococcus saccharolyticus
V. paryula	Veillonella paryula	

Clostridia

ABBREVIATION	ORGANISM	SYNONYM/OTHER DESIGNATION
C. barati	Clostridium barati	Clostridium paraperfringens
C. bifermentans	Clostridium bifermentans	
C. butyricum	Clostridium butyricum	

ABBREVIATION	ORGANISM	SYNONYM/OTHER DESIGNATION
C. cadaveris	Clostridium cadaveris	Clostridium capitovale
C. clostridioforme	Clostridium clostridioforme	Bacteroides clostridioforme
C. difficile	Clostridium difficile	
C. histolyticum	Clostridium histolyticum	
C. innocuum	Clostridium innocuum	
C. perfringens	Clostridium perfringens	
C. ramosum	Clostridium ramosum	
C. septicum	Clostridium septicum	
C. sordellii	Clostridium sordellii	
C. sporogenes	Clostridium sporogenes	
C. subterminale	Clostridium subterminale	
C. tertium	Clostridium tertium	
C. tetani	Clostridium tetani	

Anaerobic Non–Spore-forming Gram-Negative Bacilli (NSF-GNB)

ABBREVIATION	ORGANISM	SYNONYM/OTHER DESIGNATION
Bac. distasonis	Bacteroides distasonis	Bacteroides fragilis, subsp. distasonis
Bac. eggerthii	Bacteroides eggerthii	
Bac. fragilis	Bacteroides fragilis	Bacteroides fragilis, subsp. fragilis
Bac. ovatus	Bacteroides ovatus	Bacteroides fragilis, subsp. ovatus
Bac. thetaiota	Bacteroides thetaiotaomicron	Bacteroides fragilis, subsp. thetaiotaomicron
Bac. uniformis	Bacteroides uniformis	
Bac. ureolyticus	Bacteroides ureolyticus	Bacteroides corrodens
Bac. vulgatus	Bacteroides vulgatus	Bacteroides fragilis, subsp. vulgatus
Capnocytopha sp.	Capnocytophaga species	D F-I; Bacteroides ochraceus
Fuso. mortiferum	Fusobacterium mortiferum	
Fuso. necrophorum	Fusobacterium necrophorum	Sphaerophorus necrophorus
Fuso. nucleatum	Fusobacterium nucleatum	Fusobacterium fusiforme
Fuso. varium	Fusobacterium varium	
Pre. bivia	Prevotella bivia	Bacteroides bivius
Pre. buccae	Prevotella buccae	Bacteroides buccae
Pre. corporis	Prevotella corporis	Bacteroides corporis
Pre. disiens	Prevotella disiens	Bacteroides disiens

ABBREVIATION	ORGANISM	SYNONYM/OTHER DESIGNATION
Pre. melaninogen	Prevotella melaninogenica	Bacteroides melaninogenicus
Pre. oralis	Prevotella oralis	Bacteroides oralis
Por. asaccharolyt	Porphyromonas asaccharolytica	Bacteroides asaccharolytics
Por. gingivalis	Porphyromonas gingivalis	Bacteroides gingivalis

Anaerobic Non–Spore-forming Gram-Positive Bacilli (NSF-GPB)

ABBREVIATION	ORGANISM	SYNONYM/OTHER DESIGNATION
Act. israelii	Actinomyces israelii	
Act. odontolytic	Actinomyces odontolyticus	
Act. viscosus	Actinomyces viscosus	
Bif. dentium	Bifidobacterium dentium	
Eub. lentum	Eubacterium lentum	
Eub. limosum	Eubacterium limosum	
Lacto. sp.	Lactobacillus species	
Prop. acnes	Propionibacterium acnes	
Prop. granulosum	Propionibacterium granulosum	

HAEMOPHILUS

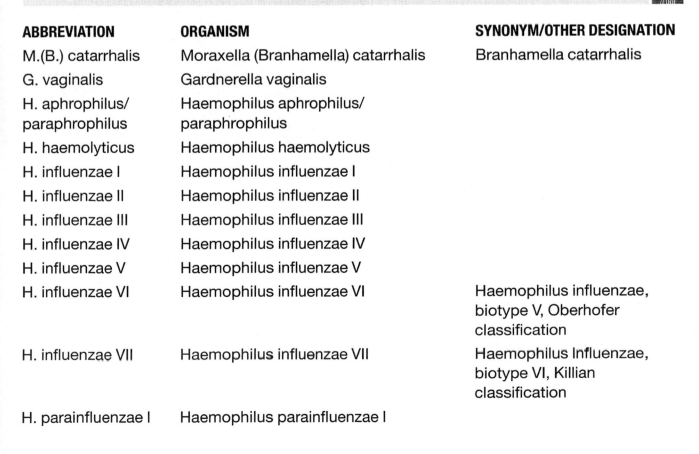

ABBREVIATION	ORGANISM	SYNONYM/OTHER DESIGNATION
M.(B.) catarrhalis	Moraxella (Branhamella) catarrhalis	Branhamella catarrhalis
G. vaginalis	Gardnerella vaginalis	
H. aphrophilus/ paraphrophilus	Haemophilus aphrophilus/ paraphrophilus	
H. haemolyticus	Haemophilus haemolyticus	
H. influenzae I	Haemophilus influenzae I	
H. influenzae II	Haemophilus influenzae II	
H. influenzae III	Haemophilus influenzae III	
H. influenzae IV	Haemophilus influenzae IV	
H. influenzae V	Haemophilus influenzae V	
H. influenzae VI	Haemophilus influenzae VI	Haemophilus influenzae, biotype V, Oberhofer classification
H. influenzae VII	Haemophilus influenzae VII	Haemophilus Influenzae, biotype VI, Killian classification
H. parainfluenzae I	Haemophilus parainfluenzae I	

ABBREVIATION	ORGANISM	SYNONYM/OTHER DESIGNATION
H. parainfluenzae II	Haemophilus parainfluenzae II	
H. parainfluenzae III	Haemophilus parainfluenzae III	
H. parainfluenzae IV	Haemophilus parainfluenzae IV	
N. gonorrhoeae	Neisseria gonorrhoeae	
N. lactamica	Neisseria lactamica	
N. meningitidis	Neisseria meningitidis	
N. mucosa (NIT+)	Neisseria mucosa (NIT+)	
Neisseria sp.	Neisseria species	

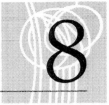

Radiology

RADIOLOGY STUDIES

NOTE: If you were transcribing the actual radiology report, you would capitalize the study. However, in general transcription, you would not capitalize the study unless it was a proper name.

abdomen flat and up decubitus

abdomen/KUB 1 view

abdominal aorta ultrasound

abdominal aortogram

abdominal biopsy

abscess drainage

acromioclavicular joint

acute abdominal series

additional views

additional views diagnostic mammogram

amniocentesis guide

angiogram pulmonary bilateral

angiogram pulmonary unilateral

angiogram selective each add vessel

angiography embolization

angiography infusion

angiography thru exist C

ankle 2 views

aorta catheter nonselective

aortogram abdominal

aortogram abdominal with runoff

aortogram thoracic

aortogram-femoral

arteriogram arch study

arteriogram carotid selective unilateral

arteriogram cerebral bilateral

arteriogram cerebral unilateral

arteriogram cervical carotid bilateral

arteriogram extremity bilateral

arteriogram extremity unilateral

arteriogram renal bilateral

arteriogram renal unilateral

arteriogram vertebral

arteriovenous fistulogram

arteriovenous shunt dialysis puncture

arthrogram elbow

arthrogram hip

arthrogram knee

arthrogram shoulder

arthrogram wrist

aspirate fluid from joint

babygram/kiddiegram

barium enema

barium enema partial limited

barium enema screening alt/colonoscopy

barium enema screening alt/sigmoidoscopy

barium enema with or without air contrast

barium swallow esophagus

barium swallow modified

bilateral diagnostic mammogram

bilateral pulmonary arteriogram

bilateral renal arteriogram

bilateral screening mammogram

bilateral selective carotid

biliary catheter exchange percutaneous

biliary dilation with or without stent

biliary drainage introducer catheter

biliary stent percutaneous dilation

biliary stent placement

biliary stone removal

biophysical profile/call reports

biopsy kidney

biopsy liver

biopsy pancreas

biopsy prostate

biopsy subcutaneous tissue

biopsy thyroid

bone age PA both hand/wrist

bone biopsy (deep)

bone biopsy (superficial)

bone gallium scan

bone scan (limited) spectrum

bone scan metastatic

bone scan—three phase

bone scan—total body

bone superficial

bone survey metabolic or traumatic

bone/skeletal survey metastatic

brain SPECT scan

breast biopsy specimen x-ray

breast biopsy stereotactic

breast biopsy ultrasound core

breast cyst aspiration

breast needle localization

C-spine FL-exterior-AB-pillar

calcium scoring

cardiovascular stress test

carotid arch

catheter introducer aorta

catheter selective abdomen pelvis 1st

catheter selective segment or subseq. PA

catheter selective thoracic additional 3rd

celiac plexus nerve block

central venous catheter by cutdown

central venous catheter percutaneous
   placement

cervical spine trauma

cervical spine with obliques

cervical spine view AP/lateral flex exterior

change gastrostomy tube

change nephrostomy tube

chest 1 view

chest 2 views—PA and lateral

chest apical lordotic 3 views

chest fluoroscopy

chest lateral decubitus

chest tube insertion

chest with obliques

cholangiogram operative

cholangiogram T tube

cholangiogram transvenous percutaneous

cisternogram imaging

clavicle

comparison film

comparison radiological consult

C-spine AP-lateral/odontoid

C-spine complete oblique—non T

CT abdominal/retroperitoneal biopsy

CT angiogram circle of Willis

CT angiogram of chest for dissection

CT angiogram of chest for pulmonary embolus

CT angiogram of pelvis

CT appendiceal abscess drain

CT Biomet of hip

CT biopsy guidance

CT bone biopsy (deep)

CT bone biopsy (superficial)

CT celiac plexus nerve block

CT coronal sinuses

CT for renal calculi

CT guide for stereotactic

CT limited sinuses

CT liver biopsy

CT liver biopsy with major procedure

CT liver drainage

CT lung abscess drainage

CT lung biopsy

CT lymph node biopsy

CT lymph node drainage

CT maxillofacial with or without contrast

CT muscle biopsy

CT of angiogram of abdomen

CT of angiogram carotids

CT of brain with or without contrast

CT of cervical spine with or without contrast

CT of chest with or without contrast

CT of chest with or without contrast (limited)

CT of lower extremity with or without contrast

CT of lower extremity with or without contrast (limited)

CT of lumbar spine with or without contrast

CT of lumbar spine with or without contrast (limited)

CT of maxillofacial with or without contrast

CT of neck with or without contrast

CT of pelvis with or without contrast

CT of pelvis with or without contrast (limited)

CT of thoracentesis

CT of thoracentesis with tube

CT of thoracic spine with or without contrast

CT of upper extremity with or without contrast

CT or upper extremity with or without contrast (limited)

CT orbit sella-P fossa with or without contrast

CT orbits of face for fracture

CT pancreatic biopsy

CT pancreatitis drainage

CT pelvis with contrast

CT pelvis with contrast (limited)

CT pelvis with or without contrast

CT peritoneal abscess drain

CT pleura biopsy

CT radiation planning

CT reconstruction

CT renal abscess drain

CT renal biopsy

CT renal cyst aspiration

CT request for service

CT retroperitoneal abscess drainage

CT sterotactic (stealth)

CT subphrenic abscess drain

CT temporal bones with or without contrast

CT virtual colonoscopy

CVA repositioning

cystogram

cystogram in x-ray

cystogram Injection

cystourethrogram voiding

CytoGam inject

dacryocystogram

DEXA study

diagnostic radionuclides

drainage abscess/hematoma

duodenography hypotonic

each additional vessel selected

embolization non head

Enterotube placement

ERCP

esophageal dilation/dilatation

esophageal transit study

exchange drainage catheter

external biliary drainage

extremity artery

extremity ultrasound

extremity vein puncture injection

facet joint injection

facet joint injection cervical/thoracic
   additional

facet joint injection each additional level

facet joint injection lumbar/sacral

facet joint injection lumbar/sacral additional

fetal biophysical profile

fluoro 1 hour

fluoro for SI/nerve root injection

fluoro over 1 hour

fluoroscopic guidance nerve right

fluoroscopy catheter position

fluoroscopy/GI tube for position

Foley tray (no catheter)

follow-up injection/post therapy

foot 2 views

foot complete 3 views

galactogram multi ducts

galactogram single duct

gastric emptying study

GI bleed

GI bleeding study

global bilateral diagnostic mammogram

global bilateral screening mammogram

global unilateral mammogram

heel/oscalcis

Helicobacter pylori test

hepatic venography with or without
   hemodynamic evaluation

hepatobiliary imaging

hepatobiliary scan

Hexabrix 320 20 ml injection

hip 2 views child or infant

hip arthrogram

hip bilateral include pelvis

hip include pelvis

hip unilateral include pelvis

hysterosalpingogram

hysterosalpingogram injection

123 I thyroid scan and uptake

123 I thyroid uptake

I-131 thyroid therapy

inferior vena cava filter placement

inferior vena cava umbrella

inject vein

injection for myelography

injection procedure with
   hysterosalpingogram

injection procedure with sinogram

injection via nephrostomy

internal auditory canals

intraoperative ankle

intraoperative atherectomy peripheral

intraoperative atherectomy peripheral each
   additional

intraoperative atherectomy renal art

intraoperative atherectomy visceral

intraoperative atherectomy visceral
 additional

intraoperative chest

intraoperative cholangiogram

intraoperative cystogram/retrograde

intraoperative elbow

intraoperative femur

intraoperative foot

intraoperative forearm

intraoperative hand

intraoperative hip

intraoperative humerus

intraoperative intervascular ultrasound each
 additional

intraoperative intervascular ultrasound INIT ves.

intraoperative knee

intraoperative pelvis

intraoperative shoulder

intraoperative skull

intraoperative spine

intraoperative TIB/FIB

intraoperative ureteral dilation

intraoperative voiding cystourethrogram

intraoperative wrist

intravascular stent additional

introducer catheter vena cava

Isovue-M-300

IV pyelogram

IV pyelogram hypertensive

joint injection

knee 2 views

knees standing

knee with patella

knee with patella obliques

lateral cervical spine

leg length/orthoroentgenogram

LeVeen shunt

limited abdominal ultrasound

limited CAT scan

liver abscess drainage

liver biopsy

liver/spleen imaging SPECT

loopogram injection

loopogram/nephrostogram

lower extremity infant 2 views

lumbar diskogram

lumbar puncture injection

lumbar spine

lumbar spine with obliques

lung abscess drainage

lung biopsy

lung biopsy (percutaneous other)

lung or mediastinum percutaneous biopsy

lung scan perfusion

lung scan ventilation imaging only

lung scan ventilation/perfusion

lung ventilation with aerosol

lymph node biopsy—superficial

lymph node drainage

lymphangiogram bilateral

lymphangiogram injection

lymphangiogram lymphoma bilateral

lymphangiogram lymphoma unilateral

lymphatic and lymph gland imaging

mandible limited—3 views

mandible post OS series

mandible series

marking only (invasive procedure)

mastoids

Meckel's localization

Mobile Pixie bone density

mobile screening mammogram

MRA of abdomen

MRA of chest

MRA of head and neck

MRA or lower extremity

MRA of pelvis

MRA of upper extremity

MRI of abdomen

MRI of brain with brain stem

MRI of brain with or without contrast

MRI of breast bilateral

MRI of breast unilateral

MRI of cervical spine with or without contrast

MRI of chest

MRI of lower extremity

MRI of lower extremity joint

MRI of lumbar spine with or without contrast

MRI of pelvis

MRI of upper extremity

MRI orbit face, neck

MRI spectroscopy

MRI temporomandibular joints

MRI thoracic spine with or without contrast

MRI upper extremity joint

MUGA resting

MUGA (blood pool imaging) CE

muscle biopsy

myelogram cervical

myelogram lumbar

myelogram thoracic

myelogram total

myocardial infarct imaging

myocardial perfusion wall motion

nasal bones nasopharynx

neck soft tissue

needle biopsy fluoroscopy

needle introducer aorta transluminal

needle introducer retro brachial

neonatal head ultrasound

nephrostogram/loopogram

nephrostomy introducer catheter percutaneous

nephrostomy tube exchange

nephrotomography

nerve root injection cervical/thoracic

nerve root injection cervical/thoracic additional

nerve root injection each additional level

nerve root injection lumbar/sacral additional

nerve root injection single

NM stress test only

operative cholangiogram

optic foramina

orbits foreign body/fracture

pancreatic biopsy

pancreatitis drainage

Panorex mandible TMJ

parathyroid scan

pelvic angiogram

pelvic ultrasound

pelvimetry

pelvis and hips, newborn and child

per biliary drainage interior/exterior

Percufix

percutaneous dilation biliary stricture

percutaneous introducer transhepatic stent

percutaneous lung biopsy

percutaneous nephrostomy

percutaneous placement of gastro tube

percutaneous retroperitoneal drain

percutaneous stent placement

percutaneous transcatheter retrieval

percutaneous transcatheter retrieval foreign body

percutaneous transluminal angioplasty

percutaneous transluminal angioplasty aorta

percutaneous transluminal angioplasty brachiocephalic artery

percutaneous transluminal angioplasty femoral popliteal artery

percutaneous transluminal angioplasty iliac artery

percutaneous transluminal angioplasty peripheral artery

percutaneous transluminal angioplasty peripheral artery additional

percutaneous transluminal angioplasty renal/visceral artery

percutaneous transluminal angioplasty tibioperoneal artery

percutaneous transluminal angioplasty venous

percutaneous transluminal angioplasty visceral each additional

percutaneous transluminal angioplasty visceral/renal artery

percutaneous transvenous portography

percutaneous ureteral stent catheter

peritoneal abscess drain

peritoneal drainage

peritoneal ventricular shunt PAT

PET scan

physical interpretation of EKG report

physical supervision of stress

Pixie bone-density scan

pleura biopsy

portable abdomen 1 view

portable abdomen 2 views

portable ankle

portable babygram (chest and abdomen)

portable babygram/kiddiegram

portable chest 1 view

portable chest 2 views—PA and lateral

portable elbow

portable femur

portable foot

portable forearm

portable hand

portable hip 1 view

portable hip 2 views

portable humerus

portable knee

portable lumbar spine 1 view

portable pelvis

portable shoulder

portable skull

portable spine

portable spine 1 view

portable TIB/FIB lower leg

portable wrist

Port-A-Cath insertion

Port-A-Cath removal

postoperative cholangiogram

pregnancy ultrasound

prostate ultrasound

pylori breath test

radiopharmaceutical diagnostic

radiopharmaceutic therapeutic

radiopharmaceutic therapy

RBC hemangioma imaging SPECT

renal (kidney) ultrasound

renal abscess drain

renal biopsy

renal cyst aspiration

renal vein injection bilateral

renal vein renins

renal vein study

renogram with Capto or Lasix

renogram with pharmaceutical interpretation

request for service

retrograde pyelogram in cystogram

retroperitoneal abscess drainage

RFA (radiofrequency ablation study)

ribs bilateral with or without contrast

ribs unilateral with or without contrast

routine ankle 3 views

sacrococcygeal area

sacroiliac joints

scapula

scoliosis survey

scrotal ultrasound

selective catheter abdominal pelvic LE 2nd

selective catheter abdominal pelvic LE 3rd

selective catheter LR pulmonary artery

selective catheter placement venous

selective catheter placement venous 2nd

selective catheter thoracic 1st order

selective catheter thoracic 2nd order

selective catheter thoracic 3rd order

selective catheter venous sampling

sella turcica

sentinel node imaging

sentinel node mapping limited area

sentinel node mapping multiple area

sialogram

sialogram injection

sinogram/fistulogram

sinus tract injection

sinuses waters only

small bowel enteroclysis

SPECT liver scan

spinal scoliosis series

spine lateral bending

stent intravascular placement

stent placement in ureter

stereo breast biopsy guide

sternoclavicular joints

stone extraction

stress Cardiolite

stress myocardial perfusion imaging

subphrenic abscess drain

TC-thyroid scan

temporomandibular joints bilateral

temporomandibular joints unilateral

therapeutic radionuclides

thoracentesis

thoracic spine

thoracolumbar spine

thrombectomy venous axillary

thrombectomy—arteriovenous fistula

thrombectomy—venous, iliac, femoral

thrombectomy—venous/arterial graft

thyroid imaging

thyroid scan and uptake

thyroid ultrasound

thyroid uptake multi

thyroid uptake single

tibia & fibula/lower leg

TIPS hepatic venography

TIPS portal decompressed venous anast.

TIPS transluminal balloon angiogram

TMJ injection

tomogram

tomogram of kidney

transaxillary aortogram

transcatheter biopsy

transcatheter stent placement

transcatheter therapy thomb.

transcatheter vascular retrieval

transvaginal ultrasound

transvenous cholangiogram percutaneous
  injection

T-tube cholangiogram post operative

tumor/infect local

ultrasound abdomen (complete)

ultrasound abdomen limited (RUQ and LUQ)

ultrasound aorta (abdominal)

ultrasound amniocentesis

ultrasound aspiration of abscess or
  hematoma

ultrasound aspiration of liver cyst

ultrasound aspiration of pancreas cyst

ultrasound aspiration of renal cyst

ultrasound aspiration of subcutaneous
  abscess

ultrasound biopsy of kidney

ultrasound biopsy of liver

ultrasound biopsy of pancreas

ultrasound biopsy of prostate

ultrasound biopsy of thyroid

ultrasound breast

ultrasound check for fluid or marking

ultrasound extremity and effusions/hip

ultrasound guide biopsy

ultrasound guide for cyst any location

ultrasound guide paracentesis

ultrasound hip(s)/infant

ultrasound infant hips

ultrasound kidney (renal)

ultrasound limited obstetrical

ultrasound neonatal brain

ultrasound obstetrical (multiple gestations)

ultrasound obstetrics (all trimesters)

ultrasound paracentesis

ultrasound pelvic (nonobstetric)

ultrasound percutaneous aspiration of liver

ultrasound percutaneous aspiration of
  pancreas

ultrasound percutaneous aspiration of inj R

ultrasound prostate or rectal wall

ultrasound request for service

ultrasound scrotum (testes)

ultrasound spinal cord (infant)

ultrasound of subcutaneous tissue

ultrasound thoracentesis

ultrasound thyroid

ultrasound transplanted kidney (renal)

unilateral breast ultrasound

unilateral mammogram

unilateral renal arteriogram

unilateral selective carotid arteriogram

unlisted procedure, vascular injection

upper extremity infant

upper GI and small bowel

upper GI and small bowel with air contrast

upper GI series

upper GI with or without air contrast

ureteral stent int. percutaneous

ureteral stent placement

urokinase infusion

US transvaginal probe only

vein injection

venacavogram inferior

venacavogram superior

venogram bilateral

venogram nuclear medicine

venogram nuclear study

venogram phleb. bilateral

venogram phleb. unilateral

venogram unilateral

venous percutaneous transluminal
  angioplasty

vertebral intracranial only

visceral arteriogram with or without contrast flush

voiding cystourethrogram

WBC/infection local (limited)

WBC/local whole body

wrist 2 views

wrist injection

xygomatic arches

zygomatic arches

Drug Lists

COMMONLY USED DRUGS

Allergic/Antihistamine

Ana-Kit
Anaplex DM
Astelin
Atuss

Benadryl
Biohist LA

Cardec Drops DM
chlorpheniramine
Chlor-Trimeton (CTM)
Claritin RediTabs
Claritin-D
Codimal DM

Decadron
Defen-LA
dexamethasone
Dimetane
diphenhydramine
Dpipen
Dura-Vent DA

Exgest LA

Hismanal

hydroxyzine

Mescolor

naldecon
Nasalcrom
Nasonex
Norel DM, Plus

Pannaz
Patanol
Periactin
Phenergan
Poly-Histine DM
promethazine

Rondec-DM

Solu-Medrol
Sterapred

Tanafed
Tussi-12

Zyrtec

Analgesic/Narcotic

acetaminophen

Amerge (migraine)

Amigesic

Anaprox DS

APAP (Anacin)

ASA (aspirin)

Atuss

benzodiazepine

Bupap

butalbital

Cafatine

Cataflam

Cephadyn

codeine

Darvocet-N

Daypro

Demerol

diclofenac sodium

Doxaphene

Duradrin

Duragesic

Ecotrin

Endocet

Esgic

Felbatol

fentanyl

Feverall

Fioricet

Florinal

flurbiprofen

hydrocodone

hydroxyzine pamoate

ibuprofen

Imitrex

Levo-Dromoran

Levsin

Lidoderm

Lorcet

Lortab

Magsal

Medigesic

Mepergan

Midrin B58

Naprelan

naproxen

Norco

Norflex

Norgesic

Nubain

oxycodone

OxyContin

Panex

Percocet

Phrenilin Forte

Ponstel

Propacet

propoxyphene

Q-Pam

Razepam

Relafen

Roxanol

Roxicet

Roxilox

Sedapap

Serzone

Sinulin

Soma

Sonata
Stadol

Talwin
Tranxene
Tylenol #3
Tylox

Ultram

Vicodin
Vicodin ES
Vicoprofen

Xylocaine

zaleplon
Zomig

Anesthetic
Alcaine drops (eyes)

bupivacaine

Diprivan

lidocaine

Marcaine

Novocain
Nupercaine

propofol

Septocaine

Versed

Antibiotics
ABC Pak
acyclovir

amoxicillin
Amoxil
ampicillin
Ancef
Augmentin
Avelox
azithromycin

bacitracin
Bactrim
Bactroban Cream
Benzamycin
Biaxin
Bicillin L-A, C-R

Ceclor
Cedax
cefaclor
cefazolin
cefixime
Cefotan
Ceftin
ceftriaxone
Cefzil
cephalexin
Cipro
ciprofloxacin
clarithromycin
Cleocin
clindamycin

dicloxacillin
doxycycline
Duricef
Dynabac

Ery-Tab 333

Flagyl

Floxin

Garamycin
gentamicin

Levaquin
levofloxacin

Macrobid
Macrolides
Minocin
minocycline

nitrofurantoin
Noroxin

Ofloxacin
Oxacillin

penicillin
penicillin VK
Pen-Vee K
polymyxin
Principen

Raxar
Rocephin

streptogramins
sulfasalazine
sulfathiazole
Sumycin
Suprax
Synercid

Tequin
tetracycline
TMP-SMZ (trimethoprim & sulfamethoxazole)
tobramycin
triamterene

trimethoprim sulfate
Trimox
Trovan

Veetids
Vibramycin

Zinacef
Zithromax
Z-Pak
Zyvox

Antedote
alprazolam

CroTab

epinephrine
EpiPen

Antiemetic
meclizine
metoclopramide

Phenergan
promethazine

Antifungal
Diflucan

griseofulvin

Lamisil
Loprox
Lotrisone

Mycelex
Mycostatin

Naftin
Nizoral

nystatin

recalcitrant

Antiviral
acyclovir
Aldara
amantadine

Denavir

Famvir
Flumadine

interferon

Kaletra (HIV)

Relenza
ribavirin

Spectazole
Sporanox
Sustiva (HIV)
Symmetrel
Synagis

Tamiflu
Terazol

Valtrex
Viracept (HIV)

Ziagen (HIV)

Antiinflammatory
Ansaid
Anturane
Arava
Arthrotec

Cataflam
Celebrex
Celestone
Clinoril

D.A. Chewtabs
Depo-Medrol
diclofenac

Enbrel

Flonase
Flovent

ibuprofen
indomethacin

ketoprofen

Lodine

Medrol Dos-Pak
methylprednisolone
Motrin

Naprosyn
naproxen
neomycin

Oruvail

prednisone
Prelone

Relafen

Tolectin
triamcinolone

Vioxx

Antineoplastic/Antinuclear

adriamycin
Alkeran
Aromasin

Casodex
Cytoxan

Ellence

fluorouracil

leucovorin
Leukeran
Lupron

Nolvadex

Oncovin

Pacis

tamoxifen citrate
Targretin
Temodar
Trelstar Depot

Viadur

Zadaxin
Zonegran

Baby: Formula

Alimentum
Alsoy

Carbofed
Carnation GoodStart

Enfamil

Isomil DF

Karo Syrup

LactAid
LactoFree

Neocate
Nutramigen

Pregestimil
ProSobee

Similac

Baby: Shots

DTaP

HBV
HIB (flu)
HIB-C

IPV (polio)

MMR (measles, mumps, rubella)

Baby: Skin

Basis

Cafcit
Cetaphil

Dove

Elocon Cream

Keri Lotion

Lubriderm

Nystatin Cream

Purpose

Baby: Miscellaneous

Mylicon Drops

Orajel (teething)

Poly-Vi-Sol Drops

Cardiovascular

Accupril

acebutolol

Aceon

Adalat CC

Adenocard

Aggrenox

Aldactone

Aldomet

Altace

amiodarone

amlodipine

Angiomax

Atacand

atenolol

Avalide

Avapro

benazepril

Betapace

Bumex

Calan

Capozide

captopril

Cardizem

Cardura

Cartia XT

chlorothiazide

chlorthalidone

cholestyramlne

clonidine

Colestid

Cordarone

Coreg

Corgard

Corzide

Coumadin

Covera

Demadex

digoxin

dihydropteridine

Dilacor

diltiazem

Diovan

dipyridamole

Dyazide

DynaCirc

felodipine

furosemide

gemfibrozil

hydrochlorothiazide

HydroDIURIL

Hygroton

Hyzaar

Imdur

integrelin

Isoptin

isosorbide

labetalol

Lanoxin

Lasix

Lescol

Lipitor

lisinopril

Lopid
Lopressor
Lotensin
Lotrel
lovastatin
Lovenox

Mavik
Maxzide
metoprolol
Mevacor
Micardis
Micro-K
Microzide
Monopril

nadolol
nifedipine
nitroglycerin
NitroQuick
Nitrostat
Normodyne
Norvasc

pindolol
Plavix
Plendil
Pravachol
prazosin
Prinivil
Prinzide
procainamide
Procardia XL
propranolol

Questran
Quinaglute
Quinidex
Quinora

Rezulin
Rythmol

Sectral
sodium morrhuate
sotalol
spironolactone
Sular

Tarka
Tenex
Tenoretic
Tenormin
terazosin
Teveten
Tiazac
Tikosyn
TNKase
Toprol
Trental
triamterene
Tridil

Univasc

Vaseretic
Vasotec
Vazosan
verapamil
Verelan
Viagra

warfarin

Zaroxolyn
Zestoretic
Zestril
Ziac
Zocor

Dermatologic

Abreva

Accutane

Aclovate Cream

Acticin

Acute Derm Anti-Acne Kit

Aldara

Aloe Vera Gel

AmLactin

Analpram

Anusol

Aristocort

Atarax

Aveeno Product

Bactroban Cream

Balmex

Benzac

Benzamycin

Benzoin

Caladryl

Capsaicin Cream

Celestoderm

Celestone

Cleocin

Cloderm Cream

Cortate

cortisone

Cortizone

Desenex

Diprolene

docosanol

Dynacin

Efudex

Eldoquin Forte

Elimite

Elocon

erythromycin

Eucerin

Exsel

Flanders Ointment

Fucidin

Furacin

Granulex Spray

hydrocortisone

hydroquinone

Kenalog

Klout

Kwell

Lac-Hydrin

LactAid

Lamisil

Lidex Cream

Loprox

Lotrimin

Lotrisone

Mentax

MetroGel

MetroLotion

Minoxidil

Mederma

Mycolog

Mytrex Cream

Neosporin

Nizoral

Nystatin

Oxistat

Pancrease

Permethrin

Phenol

Propecia

Psorcon

Renova

Retin-A

Rogaine

Salactic Film

Salicylic Acid

Santyl

Sarna Lotion

Silvadene Cream

Spectazole

Sporanox

Tazorac Cream

Temovate Preparations

Topicort

triamcinolone

trichloroacetic acid

Tridesilon

triple antibiotic ointment

Ultravate

Unasyn

Vytone

Westcort Cream

Zetar

Zostrix Cream

Endocrine: Diabetes

Actos

Amaryl

Avandia

DiaBeta

Diabinese

glipizide

GlucaGen

Glucophage

Glucotrol XL

glyburide

Glynase

Humalog

Humulin

Lantus, Lantuss

metformin

Micronase

Novolin

NovoLog

NPH Insulin

Orinase

Prandin

Precose

Rezulin

Starlix

tolazamide

Tolinase

Ultralente

Ultrase

Velosulin BR

Endocrine: Thyroid

Cytomel

Hectorol

Levothroid
levothyroxine
Levoxyl

propylthiouracil

Synthroid

Tapazole

Endocrine: Miscellaneous
Androderm
AndroGel

Nutropin Depot

Proscar

Gastrointestinal
acidophilus
Aciphex
Actigall
Asacol
Axid

Bentyl
bethanechol

Carafate
cimetidine
Citrucel
Colace

dexamphetamine
Donnatal

Emetrol

famotidine
FiberCon

Flomax

Gaviscon
GoLYTELY

Helidac
hyoscyamine

lactulose
Lariam
Levbid
Levsin
Levsinex
Librax
Lomotil
loperamide
Lotronex

Maalox
magnesium oxide
Maltsupex
meclizine
Metamucil
Miralax
Mylicon

omeprazole
oxybutynin

Pepcid
Peri-Colace
perphenazine
phenazine
Phenergan
Plaquenil
Prevacid
Prevpac
Prilosec
Proctofoam HC

promethazine
Propulsid
Protonix

ranitidine
Reglan
Rowasa

Senokot
simethicone

Tagamet
Tebamide
Tigan
Torecan
Trimpex

Vermox

Zantac
Zofran

Genitourinary
allopurinol
Azo-Standard

Bactrim

chlorthalidone
Cipro
Compazine
Cytotec

Detrol
Ditropan

Flomax

Macrobid
Macrodantin

nitrofurantoin

phenazopyridine
probenecid
Pyridium

saw palmetto
spironolactone

terazosin
triampyzine sulfate
triamterene

Urised
Urispas
Uristat

Viagra

Gynecologic
Alora
Antagon

C.E.S.
Cenestin
Cleocin Vaginal Cream
Climara
Clomid
CombiPatch
Cycrin

Depo-Provera
Didronel
doxycycline
Dyazide

E2 III
Estrace
Estraderm Patch
estradiol
Estratab
Estratest
estrogen

Eulexin

Evista

FemPatch

Femstat

Flagyl

folic acid

Fosamax

medroxyprogesterone

Menest

Methergine

MetroGel

metronidazole

Miacalcin

Monistat

Mycelex

Mycostatin

M-Zole 3

Ogen

Ortho-Est

Ortho-Prefest

Ovidrel

oxytocin

phytoestrogen

Precare

Premarin

Premphase

Prempro

progesterone

Prometrium

Provera

Stuart Natal Plus 3

Terazol

Valtrex

Vivelle

Vivelle-Dot

Gynecologic: Contraceptive

Alessa

Cyclessa

Demulen

Depo-Provera

Desogen

Estrostep Fe

Levlen

Levlite

Lo/Ovral

Loestrin

Microgestin Fe

Micronor

Mircette

Necon

Nordette

Norplant

Ortho Dialpak

Ortho Tri-Cyclen

Ortho-Cept

Ortho-Novum 7/7/7

Plan B

Tri-Levlen

Triphasil

Head: Cold Symptoms and Throat Ailments

Advil Sinus

albuterol metered dose inhaler

albuterol syrup

Allegra D

amoxicillin

Amoxil

Anatuss DM

Astelin Nasal Spray

Atuss

Augmentin

Benadryl

Benylin DM

benzonatate

Biaxin

Bromfed

Cardec DM

Ceftin

Cepacol

Chloraseptic

Claritin-D

Codiclear DH

Comtrex

Contuss

Debrox

Delsym

dextromethorphan

Dimetapp

Donatussin

Donnatal

Drixoral

Duratuss

Dynabac

echinacea

E.E.S.

erythromycin

Exgest

Exgest LA

Fenesin

Flonase

Guaifed-PD

guaifenesin

Guaifenex

Guaimax

Guiatuss

Guiatuss DAC

Histinex DM

Histussin-HC

Humibid DM

Hycodan

Hycomine

Hycotuss

Keflex

Lorabid

minocycline

monocycline

Muco-Fen

Muco-Fen-DM

Muco-Fen-LA

Mycelex Oral Troche

Naldelate

Nalex A

Nalex DF

Nalex DH

Nasacort

Nasarel

Nasatab

Nasonex

Neo-Synephrine

NyQuil

Ornade
Otrivin

Palgic DS
Panmist S
Pannaz
Pediazole
Phazyme
phenylpropanolamine
Privine
Profen
Profen II
Prolex DH
Protuss
Protuss DM
pseudoephedrine
P-V-Tussin

Robitussin
Robitussin DM
R-Tannate
Ru-Tuss
Rynatan

Septra
Simprex-D
Sudafed
Suprax

Tavist-D
Tessalon Perles
Tussi-12
Tussionex
Tussionex Penn Kinetic

Vancenase Nasal Spray
Vantin

Zephrex
Zyrtec

Head: Ears
Americaine
Auralgan

Cefzil
Cerumenex
Ciloxan
Coly-Mycin
Cortan B Otic
Cortisporin Otic

Debrox

Otic HC

Pediotic
Primsol Solution

Swim-Ear

VoSol HC

Zoto HC

Head: Ophthalmology
Acular Drops
Alcaine Drops
Alomide
Alphagan
Azopt

Betagan
Betoptic
Bleph-10

Ciloxan
ciprofloxacin
Crolom
Cyclogyl

Diamox

Emadine

fluorescein stain

Gantrisin
Garamycin
Genoptic
Gentak

Ilotycin

mydriatic

Naphcon-A

Ocuflox
Ophthetic

Patanol
pilocarpine
Polytrim
proparacaine

Rescula

Sodium Sulamyd

Terramycin
tetracaine
Timoptic
TobraDex

Visudyne
Vitravene

Xalatan

Hematologic
Aceon
Agrylin
AquaMEPHYTON
ardeparin

CellCept
Chromagen
Coumadin

dalteparin

enoxaparin
epoetin alfa

Ferrlecit
ferrous sulfate

Hemocyte

nadroparin
Nascobal
Neoral
Niferex
Nu-Iron

pentoxifylline
Pletal
pravastatin

Refludan

Ticlid
tinzaparin
Tricor

Zocor

Immunologic
cyclosporin

polystyrene

Musculoskeletal and Neuromuscular
Actimmune
Activelle
Actonel

Allopurinol
Anaprox DS
Anectine

baclofen

carisoprodol
Celebrex
chlorzoxazone
chondroitin sulfate
colchicine

Deltasone
diazepam

Evista

Flexeril
Fosamax

glucosamine sulfate

Imuran
Indocin

levodopa

Meclomen
Mestinon
methocarbamol
methotrexate
Miacalcin
Mobic

Naprelan

Parafon Forte
Parlodel
prednisolone
prednisone

Raplon

Robaxin

selegiline
Sinemet
Skelaxin
Supartz
Synvisc

Tasmar
Therafectin
Toradol
Trilisate

Vioxx
Voltaren XR

Zanaflex
Zyloprim

Nutritional
Calcitrol
Chromagen

KCL-20
K-Dur
K-Lor
K-tab
Klor-Con

lecithin

Os-Cal

Poly-Vi-Sol Drops

Rocaltrol

Trinsicon

Nutritional: Diet Aid
Acutrim
Adipex

Bontril

dextroamphetamine

Fastin

Ionamin

Metabolife

phentermine

Xenical

Psychiatric and Central Nervous System (CNS)

Activan
Adderall
alprazolam
Ambien
amitriptyline
Artane
atropine

bupropion
BuSpar

Celexa
cisapride
clonazepam
Cogentin
Compazine
Comtan
Copaxone
Cylert

Depakote
Desyrel
dexamphetamine
Diamox

diazepam
Dilantin
doxepin
droperidol

Effexor-XR
Elavil
Eldepryl

fluvoxamine maleate

Haldol
hydroxyzine

imipramine pamoate
Impromen
Inapsine

Keppra
Klonopin

Lamictal
levodopa
Librium
Limbitrol
lorazepam
Luvox

Mellaril
mepazine
Metadate ER
methylphenidate
Mysoline

Neurontin
nortriptyline
Novantrone

oxazepam

Pamelor

Paxil

Permax

phenobarbital

phenothiazine

Prolixin

Prozac

Raplon

Remeron

Restoril

Risperdal

Ritalin

Sarafem

Serax

Serzone

Sinequan

sodium pentobarbital

sodium phenobarbital

Stelazine

Symmetrel

Tebamide

Tegretol

temazepam

thioridazine

Tofranil

tomoxetine

Torecan

trazodone

Trilafon

Trileptal

Valium

Vistaril

Pulmonary and Asthma

Accolate

AeroBid

albuterol

Alupent

Atrovent

Avelox

Azmacort

Beclovent

Benadryl

Brethaire

Brethine

Bronkaid Mist

Combivent Inhaler

cromolyn sodium

DuoNeb

dyphylline

Entex LA

ephedrine

Florinef

Flovent

Guaifed

Guaifenex

Intal

ipratropium

isoniazid

Lodrane

Maxair

MDI—metered-dose inhaler

methacholine

Metussin

OptiChamber

Pediapred
Prelone
Primatene Mist
Proventil
Pulmicort Turbuhaler

Rocephin

Salbutamol Sulfate
Serevent
Singulair
Sterapred DS
Sterapred Unipak
Sudanyl

terbutaline
Theo-Dur
Theolair
theophylline
Tilade
Tomalate
Tussend
Tussi-Organidin DM

Uniphyl

Vanceril
Vanceril DS
Ventolin
Volmax

Xopenex

Zagam
Zyflo

Smoking Cessation
Habitrol

Nicoderm
Nicorette
Nicorette DS
nicotine bitartrate
nicotine polacrilex
Nicotrol
Nicotrol NS

Diabetic Supplies

Bayer
DEX No-Strip Testing System

Glucometer DEX Blood Glucose Monitoring
  System
Glucometer Elite blood glucose meter
Glucometer Elite XL Diabetes Care System
B-D Insulin Syringes
29-gauge, 30-gauge short
3/10 cc, 1/2 cc, 1 cc
Choice needle-free insulin injector
Ultra-Fine, II
Johnson & Johnson Lifescan
Fast Take
One Touch diabetes test strips
One Touch Basic
One Touch Penlet Plus
One Touch Profile
SureStep
MediSense
Precision Q-I-D blood glucose monitor
Precision Sure-Dose
Precision Xtra
Roche
Accu-Check Simplicity
Accu-Chek Advantage Diabetes Care Kit
Accu-Chek Complete Monitor

COMMONLY CONFUSED DRUG NAMES

Acular—Acthar
Adderall—Inderal
Adeflor—Aldoclor
adriamycin—Idamycin
albuterol—atenolol
alfentanil—Anafranil
amitriptyline—nortriptyline
Anafranil—enalapril
Anturane—Artane
Apresoline—Apresazide
Aricept—Aerosept
Asacol—Os-Cal
aspirin—Afrin
Ativan—Ativane
Atrovent—Alupent
Aventyl—Ambenyl
Avonex—Avelox
azathioprine—Azulfidine

Bactrim—bacitracin
Bentyl—Aventyl
Benylin—Ventolin
Betagan—Betagen
Bicillin—Wycillin
Brevoxyl—Benoxyl
butalbital—butabarbital

Cardene SR—Cardizem SR
Cardura—K-Dur
carteolol—carvedilol
Cartrol—Carbatrol
Catapres—Cetapred
Catapres—Combipres
cefamandole—cefmetazole
Ceftin—Cefotan
Chorex—Chymex
Cidex—Lidex

cisplatin—carboplatin
Citracal—Citrucel
Clinoril—Clozaril
Clinoril—Elavil
clonazepam—lorazepam
clonidine—Klonopin
Combipres—Catapres
Comvax—Recombivax
Coumadin—Kemadrin
Cytoxan—Ciloxan

desipramine—imipramine
desoximetasone—dexamethasone
Desoxyn—digoxin
Dexedrine—dextran
DiaBeta—Zebeta
Diamox—Trimox
digoxin—doxepin
Diprosone—dapsone
Donnagel—Donnatal
dopamine—dobutamine
Doxidan—digoxin
Doxy—Doxil
Dyazide—diazoxide

Ecotrin—Edecrin
Efidac—Efudex
Elavil—Mellaril
Eldepryl—enalapril
Epogen—Neupogen
erythromycin—azithromycin
Esimil—Estinyl
Esimil—Ismelin
Eurax—Serax
Eurax—Urex
Evoxac—Eurax

Humalog—Humulin

Hycodan—Hycomine

Hycodan—Vicodin

hydralazine—hydroxyzine

hydrochlorothiazide — hydroflumethiazide

hydroxyprogesterone—
   medroxyprogesterone

Hygroton—Regroton

Hytone—Vytone

imipenem—Omnipen

Imuran—Elmiron

interferon alfa-2b—interferon alfa-2a

Interleukin-2—interferon 2

iodine—Iopidine

isoflurane—enflurane

Isoptin—Intropin

Isordil—isuprel

Kaochlor—K-Lor

Kefzol—Cefzil

lactose—lactulose

lorazepam—alprazolam

Mellaril—Mebaral

Mephyton—melphalan

Mephyton—mephenytoin

mepivacaine—bupivacaine

mesantoin—Mestinon

Mestinon—Metatensin

methicillin—mezlocillin

methionine—methenamine

metipranolol—metaproterenol

Mevacor—Mivacron

Micro-K—Micronase

Micronase—Micronor

Midrin—Mydfrin

Mifeprex—Mirapex

Minocin—Mithracin

Minocin—niacin

Moban – Mobidin

Mycelex—Myoflex

naldecon—Nalfon

Patanol—Platinol

Pathocil—Placidyl

Paxil—Doxil

Pediapred—Pediazole

penicillamine—penicillin

Pentax—Penetrex

Pentax—Permax

pentobarbital—phenobarbital

pentosan—pentostatin

Perative—Periactin

Percocet—Percodan

Permax—Pernox

peroxyl—Benoxyl

phenytoin—mephenytoin

pindolol—Panadol

Platinol—pindolol

Plendil—Pletal

Posicor—Proscar

prednisolone—prednisone

Premarin—Remeron

Restoril—Vistaril

Retrovir—ritonavir

ribavirin—riboflavin

rimantadine—ranitidine

ritodrine—ranitidine

Roxicet—Roxanol

Serax—Xerac

Serophene—Sarafem

sertraline—Serentil

Slo-bid—Dolobid

Slow FE—Slow-K

somatropin—somatrem

sotalol—Stadol

sufentanil—alfentanil

sulfasalazine—sulfadiazine

Suprax—Sporanox

Surbex—Carbex

Surfak—Surbex

Taxol—Paxil

Tenex— Entex

Vanceril—Vansil

Vasosulf—Velosef

Ventolin—Benylin

Ventolin—Vantin

Verelan—Virilon

vinblastine—vincristine

Vioxx—Zyvox

Volmax—Flomax

Voltaren—Verelan

Vytone—Hytone

Wellferon—warfarin

Xalatan—Travatan

Xanax—Tenex

Xanax—Xopenex

Zestril—Restoril

Zocor—Cozaar

Zofran—Zosyn

Zovirax—Zostrix

Zyloprim—ZORprin

10

Confusing Words, Abbreviations, and Eponyms

COMMONLY MISUSED WORDS

abduct	flex away
adduct	flex inward
accept	receive willingly
except	exclude
advice	an opinion
advise	to give an opinion
a febrile	increased fever
afebrile	without fever
affect	psychological disposition; action word (e.g., affecting activities of daily living, flat affect)
effect	result (e.g., drug side effect)
allusion	casual mention
elusion	evading something
illusion	misleading appearance
Ansaid	name brand medication (antiinflammatory)
NSAID	nonsteroidal antiinflammatory drug
anonymous	unidentified
unanimous	unified
apposition	bringing two parts together
opposition	act of conflict against

anterior	pertaining to front part
interior	pertaining to inside part
inferior	pertaining to the lesser part
arrhythmia	irregular heartbeat
erythema	redness
aural	pertaining to the ears
oral	pertaining to the mouth
carotene	yellowish chemical pigment
keratin	protein found in teeth, nails, and skin
censor	to edit
censure	to reprimand
cite	a notation
site	a location
sight	vision
climatic	pertaining to the weather
climactic	pertaining to climax
coarse	rough, thick
course	pathway
complement	complete
compliment	praise, flatter
conscience	sense of moral standards (right and wrong)
conscious	state of being awake and alert
cord	thick string (spinal cord)
chord	a group of strings that produces sound
cystalgic	pertaining to bladder pain
systolic	pertaining to the heartbeat
cytology	cell biology
sitiology	study of dietetics

decision	a choice
discission	an incision
discoid	disk-like
discord	not agreeing; conflict
defuse	make nonfunctional
diffuse	spread out
discreet	to discern; lacking pretension; reserved speech
discrete	constituting a separate thing; unconnected distinct parts
descent	going down
dissent	disagree
ductal	pertaining to channel
ductile	flexible
dysphagia	difficulty swallowing
dysphasia	difficulty speaking
elicit	cause
illicit	illegal
emanate	come from
eminent	prominent
enervation	weakening
innervation	distribution of nerves
innovation	new method
etiology	cause
ideology	study of ideas
explicit	distinct; not vague
implicit	implied
facial	pertaining to the face
fascial	pertaining to fibrous tissue
farther	extra distance
further	additional amount

fascicular	relating to muscle fibers (cardiac, fascicular block)
vesicular	relating to a vesicle (bladder-like, blister)
flanges	dental edges
phalanges	fingers, toes
gauge	measurement
gouge	scoop out
heal	to restore health
heel	round posterior portion of the posterior foot; behind the ankle
hill	incline smaller than a mountain
idle	inactive
idol	symbol of worship
ileum	intestine
ilium	hip
it's	contraction for *it is*
its	possessive for belonging to it
knuckle	dorsal aspect of the phalangeal joint
nuchal	pertaining to the neck
labile	constantly shifting
labial	pertaining to the lips
later	subsequent time
latter	most recent to two previously named items
lay	to place
lie	untruth; to deceive or recline
led	past tense of the verb to lead
lead	chemical element; to guide a direct course
liable	accountable
libel	defamatory comment
lichen	plant formed of fungus; algae
liken	to compare

loop	cord-like structure
loupe	magnifying lens
loose	not tight
lose	to misplace or to be defeated
manor	estate
manner	socially correct; a way of doing something, behavior
meiosis	cell division
miosis	constriction of pupils
melitis	cheek inflammation
mellitus	metabolic disease (e.g., diabetes mellitus)
myelitis	spinal cord inflammation
moral	ethical
morale	mood
mucous	adjective of mucus (e.g., mucous membranes are clear)
mucus	noun form of mucus (e.g., clear mucus noted)
osteal	bony
ostial	opening into a tubular organ or between two body cavities
packed	bundled
pact	agreement
palpation	examination of feeling by fingers
palpitation	throbbing
paracytic	lying among cells
parasitic	pertaining to a parasite
passed	went by; ceased
past	a former time
pediculous	infested by lice
pediculus	stem-like structure
penile	pertaining to a penis
penal	law enforcement system

perennial	lasting for many years
perineal	pertaining to the pelvic floor
peroneal	outer side of the leg
perfusion	pouring through
profusion	an abundance
personal	private; relating to a particular person
personnel	body of people employed by an organization
petal	leaf-like part
pedal	pertaining to the foot
plain	simple
plane	flat surface of a three-dimensional object
precede	before
proceed	continue; carry on an act or process
principal	primary or head
principle	rule or law
prostate	gland that surrounds the male bladder
prostrate	to overcome; to lie flat
psychosis	mental disorder
sycosis	hair follicle inflammation
pupal	pertaining to second stage of an insect
pupil	black center of the iris of the eye
radical	extreme (e.g., radical mastectomy)
radicle	a small root
rational	logical
rationale	justification
reflex	involuntary movement
reflux	backward flow
regimen	scheme for diet or exercise
regiment	Army division; of strict control
regime	political system

retrocolic	pertaining to the colon
retrocollic	pertaining to the back of the neck
right	direction; correct
write	to record
root	embedded part or cause
route	path
rye	grain
wry	twisted or bent (e.g., wry neck)
sac	pouch-like
sack	bag
saccharin	artificial sweetener
saccharine	pertaining to sugar
sail	object on a boat that catches the wind
sale	availability of goods for purchase; may be at a lower cost
sell	to surrender goods for money
cell	smallest structure of an organism; small room of confinement
scatoma	fecal matter in colon
scotoma	depressed vision in visual field
scirrhous	hard
cirrhosis	liver disease
scirrhus	carcinoma
serous	containing serum
serious	important matter
set	to place something
sit	to rest
soar	to fly
sore	tender to touch
stationary	immovable
stationery	paper

| their | possessive; belonging to |
| there | place |

to	in the direction of
too	also; more than enough
two	Arabic number 2

| trophic | nutrition |
| tropic | change |

| vesical | bladder |
| vesicle | small sac containing liquid |

| viscous | thick; syrupy |
| viscus | large organ |

| waive | to relinquish or forgo |
| wave | a hand greeting |

| who's | contraction for *who is* |
| whose | that which belongs to whom |

| your | possessive form of you |
| you're | contraction for *you are* |

COMMONLY USED MEDICAL ABBREVIATIONS

AAMT	American Association for Medical Transcriptionists
AB	number of aborted fetuses
ABG	arterial blood gas
ACL	anterior cruciate ligament
ACNP	Acute Care Nurse Practitioner
AD	right ear
ADA	American Diabetes Association
AKA	above-knee amputation
	also known as
AMA	American Medical Association
	against medical advice
ANA	antinuclear antibody
A & P	anterior and posterior
	auscultation and percussion
	assessment and plan

AS	left ear
ASAP	as soon as possible
ASCVD	arteriosclerotic cardiovascular disease
AU	both ears
BBB	bundle branch block
BCP	birth control pills
BE	barium enema
BKA	below-knee amputation
BP	blood pressure
BPD	biparietal diameter
	bronchopulmonary dysplasia
BPH	benign prostatic hypertrophy
BRAT diet	bananas, rice, applesauce, and toast diet
BSER	brain stem–evoked response
BUN	blood urea nitrogen
BUS	Bartholin's, urethral, and Skene's glands
CA	carcinoma
CABG	coronary artery bypass graft (dictated as cabbage)
CAT	computerized axial tomography
CBC	complete blood count
CEA	carcinoembryonic antigen
CHD	congestive heart disease
CHF	congestive heart failure
CIWA-Ar	Clinical Institute Withdrawal Assessment for Alcohol-revised (dictated as "see-wa")
CNS	central nervous system
COPD	chronic obstructive pulmonary disease
CPAP	continuous positive airway pressure
CPD	cephalopelvic disproportion
CPR	cardiopulmonary resuscitation
	computerized patient record
C & S	culture and sensitivity
CSF	cerebrospinal fluid
CT	computerized tomography
CVA	cerebrovascular accident
	costovertebral angle

D & C	dilation and curettage
DDD	degenerative disk disease
DEXA	dual-energy x-ray absorptiometry
DJD	degenerative joint disease
DO	doctor of osteopathy
DOA	dead on arrival
DOE	dyspnea on exertion
DPT	diphtheria, pertussis, and tetanus (immunization)
DTRs	deep tendon reflexes
ECG	electrocardiogram
ECHO	echocardiogram
ECT	electroconvulsive therapy
ED	Emergency Department
EDC	estimated date of confinement
EEG	electroencephalogram
EG	esophagogastric
EGD	esophagogastroduodenoscopy
EKG	electrocardiogram
EMG	electromyography
EMR	electronic medical record
EMS	Emergency Medical Service
ENG	electronystagmography
ENT	ears, nose, and throat
EOMI	extraocular movement/motion intact
ER	emergency room
ESP	extrasensory perception
ESR	erythrocyte sedimentation rate
EST	electroshock treatment
ET	endotracheal
ETOH	ethanol, alcohol
FB	foreign body
FBS	fasting blood sugar
FSH	follicle-stimulating hormone
G	gravida
GC	gonococcus

GENT	gentamicin (drug)
GERD	gastroesophageal reflux disease
GI	gastrointestinal
GU	genitourinary
GYN	gynecology
HBV	hepatitis B vaccine/virus
hCG	human chorionic gonadotropin (blood pregnancy test)
HCT	hematocrit
HEENT	head, eyes, ears, nose, and throat
HGB	hemoglobin
H & H	hemoglobin and hematocrit
HIB	Haemophilus influenza B (vaccine)
HIB-C	Haemophilus influenza B (vaccine) conjugate
HIPAA	Health Insurance Portability and Accountability Act
HIV	human immunodeficiency virus
HMO	health maintenance organization
H & P	history and physical
HPI	history of present illness
IAC	internal auditory canal
ICU	Intensive Care Unit
I & D	incision and drainage
IM	intramuscular
INR	international normal rate
I & O	intake and output
IPPB	intermittent positive-pressure breathing
IQ	intelligence quotient
IU	international units
IUD	intrauterine device
IV	intravenous
IVP	intravenous pyelogram
JVD	jugular venous distention
KOH	potassium hydroxide
KUB	kidneys, ureters, and bladder
LIMA	left internal mammary artery (dictated as "leema")
LLL	left lower lobe

LLQ	left lower quadrant
LMP	last menstrual period
LS	lumbosacral
LUL	left upper lobe
LUQ	left upper quadrant
MCP	metacarpophalangeal joint
MD	medical doctor
MI	myocardial infarction
MMR	mumps, measles, and rubella (immunization)
MRI	magnetic resonance imaging
MRSA	methicillin-resistant Staphylococcus aureus (dictated as "marsa")
MS	multiple sclerosis
NG	nasogastric
NKA	no known allergies
NPH	isophane insulin
NPO	nothing by mouth
NSAIDs	nonsteroidal antiinflammatory drug
NST	nonstress test
OB	obstetrics
OBS	organic brain syndrome
OCD	obsessive-compulsive disorder
OD	right eye
O & P	ova and parasites
OR	operating room
ORIF	open reduction and internal fixation
OS	left eye
OTC	over-the-counter
OU	both eyes
P	para (live births)
PA	posteroanterior
	Physician's Assistant
PA-C	Physician's Assistant-Certified
PAC	premature atrial contractions
PAT	paroxysmal atrial tachycardia

PCN	penicillin
PCP	primary care physician
PE	peripheral edema
	pleural effusion
	pharyngoesophageal
	physical examination
	pulmonary embolus
PEEP	positive end-expiratory pressure
PERLA	pupils equal and reactive to light and accommodation
PID	pelvic inflammatory disease
PMH	past medical history
PMI	point of maximum impulse
PND	paroxysmal nocturnal dyspnea
PR	per rectum
PROM	premature rupture of membranes
	passive range of motion
PSA	prostate-specific antigen
PTA	prior to admission
PVC	premature ventricular contractions
QA	quality assurance
QS	sufficient quantity
RBC	red blood cell
	red blood count
REM	rapid eye movement
RLL	right lower lobe
RLQ	right lower quadrant
R/O	rule out
ROS	review of systems
RSD	reflex sympathetic dystrophy
RUL	right upper lobe
RUQ	right upper quadrant
SAB	spontaneous abortion
SC	subcutaneous
SCM	sternocleidomastoid
SH	social history

SI	sacroiliac
SIDS	sudden infant death syndrome
SMAC	superior mesenteric artery count
SR	sedimentation rate
	sinus rhythm
SSS	sick sinus syndrome
STD	sexually transmitted disease
T & A	tonsillectomy and adenoidectomy
TAB	therapeutic abortion
TAH-BSO	total abdominal hysterectomy/bilateral salpingo-oophorectomy
TB	tuberculosis
TENS unit	transcutaneous electrical nerve stimulation device
TIA	transient ischemic attack
TM	tympanic membrane
TMJ	temporomandibular joint
TSH	thyroid-stimulating hormone
TURP	transurethral resection of the prostate
UA	urinalysis
UTI	urinary tract infection
UV	ureterovesical
	ultraviolet
VBAC	vaginal birth after cesarean
VD	venereal disease
VDRL	Venereal Disease Research Laboratories (lab test)
VQ scan	ventilation/perfusion lung scan
VRE	vancomycin-resistant Enterococcus
WBC	white blood cell
	white blood count
WNL	within normal limits
XRT	x-ray therapy (radiotherapy)
YO	year-old

Mixed Case Abbreviations

Bx	biopsy
Cx	cervical
	cancel
dB	decibel
Dx	diagnosis
EcoG	electrocochleogram
Fx	fracture
Hx	history
Hz	hertz
IgA	immunoglobulin A
IgD	immunoglobulin D
IgE	immunoglobulin E
IgG	immunoglobulin G
IgM	immunoglobulin M
mEq	milliequivalent
MHz/mHz	megahertz
mmHg	millimeters of mercury
mRNA	messenger ribonucleic acid
pH	potential of hydrogen
Px	prognosis
	problem
Rh	Rhesus factor in blood
Rx	recipe
	prescription
	treatment
tRNA	transfer ribonucleic acid
Tx	treatment
	tissue
	therapy

AMERICAN AND INTERNATIONAL SYMBOLS, ABBREVIATIONS, AND MEASUREMENTS

Drug Administration Abbreviations

a.c.	before meals
a.m.	morning
b.i.d.	twice a day
d.	day
g, gm	gram
gr	grain
gtt	drop
gtts	drops
h.	hour
h.s.	hour of sleep
IM	intramuscular
IV	intravenous
L	liter
p.c.	after meals
p.m.	afternoon
p.o.	by mouth
PR	per rectum
p.r.n.	as needed
q.d.*	every day
q.h.*	every hour
q.i.d.*	four times a day
q.o.d.*	every other day
q.4-6h.	every 4-6 hours
q.12h.	every 12 hours
QS	sufficient quantity
SC	subcutaneous
SL	sublingual
sub q	subcutaneous
subcu	subcutaneous

American Measurement Abbreviations

ft.	foot
gal.	gallon
ht.	height

*These are dangerous abbreviations and should not be used. They should be written out instead.

in.	inch
lb.	pound
oz.	ounce
pt.	pint
qt.	quart
tbsp.	tablespoon
tsp.	teaspoon
wt.	weight
yd.	yard

International Measurement Abbreviations

cc	cubic centimeter
cm	centimeter
dL, dl	deciliter
g	gram
kg	kilogram
L	liter
mcg	microgram
mg	milligram
mIU	milli-international unit
mm	millimeter
mL, ml	milliliter
mrad	millirad
Mu	milliunit
ng	nanogram

International Symbols

%	percent
>	greater than
<	less than
"	inch
'	foot
+	positive, plus
-	negative, minus

MEDICAL CREDENTIALS

ACNP	Acute Care Nurse Practitioner
ACRN	Aids Certified Registered Nurse
ACSW	Academy of Certified Social Workers

ACT	Assistant Chief Technologist
AIN	Assistant in Nursing
AND	Associate Degree of Nursing
ANM	Assistant Nurse Manager
ANP	Adult Nurse Practitioner
AOCN	Advanced Oncology Certified Nurse
APN	Advanced Practice Nurse (may be CNS, NP, CNM, or CRNA)
APNP	Advanced Practice Nurse Prescriber
APRN	Advanced Practice Registered Nurse
ARNP	Advanced Registered Nurse Practitioner
ARNP-BC	Advanced Registered Nurse Practice—Board Certified
ART	Accredited Records Technologist
ASN	Associate of Science in Nursing
ASPN	Associated Science of Practical Nursing
AT	Art (or Activity) Therapist
BAA	Bachelor of Applied Arts in Nursing
BAN	Bachelor of Arts in Nursing
BCD	Board Certified Diplomat
BSN	Bachelor of Science in Nursing
CAN	Certified Nurses Aid
CAPA	Certified Ambulatory PeriAnesthesia Nurse
CARN	Certified Addictions Registered Nurse
CBE	Certified Breastfeeding Educator
CCM	Certified Case Manager
CCN	Critical Care Nurse
CCRN	Certified Critical Care Registered Nurse
CCS	Certified Coding Specialist
CCT	Certified Cardiovascular Technologist
CCTC	Certified Clinical Transplant Coordinator
CDAC	Certified Drug and Alcohol Counselor
CDDN	Certified Developmental Disabilities Nurse
CDE	Certified Diabetes Educator
CDMS	Certified Disability Management Specialist
CDT-MLD	Certified Decongestive Therapist—Manual Lymphedema Drainage
CEN	Certification for Emergency Nursing
CENA	Competency Evaluated Nurse Aide

CETN	Certified Enterostomal Therapy Nurse
CFNP	Certified Family Nurse Practitioner
CGRN	Certified Gastroenterological Registered Nurse
CHES	Certified Health Education Specialist
CHN	Community Health Nurse; Certified Hemodialysis Nurse
CHPN	Certified Hospice and Palliative Care
CHT	Certified Hemodialysis Technologist; Certified Hyperbaric Technologist
CHT RN	Certified Hyperbaric Technologist Registered Nurse
CIRS	Certified Insurance Rehabilitation Specialist
CLCP	Certified Life Care Planner
CLNC	Certified Legal Nurse Consultant
CLT	Certified Lymphedema Therapist
CLT-LAN	Certified Lymphedema Therapist—Lymphology Association of North America
CMA	Cardiology Medical Assistant
CMD	Certified Medical Dosimetrist
CMT	Certified Medical Transcriptionist
CN	Clinical Nurse
CNA	Certified Nurses Aide; Certified Nursing Administration
CNAA	Certified Nursing Administration, Advanced
CNC	Clinical Nurse Consultant
CNCC(C)	Certified Nurse, Critical Care
CNM	Certified Nurse Midwife
CNMT	Certified Nuclear Medicine Technologist
CNN	Certified Nephrology Nurse
CNN(C)	Certified Nurse, Critical Care, Neuroscience
CNO	Chief Nursing Officer
CNOR	Certified Nurse Operating Room
CNRN	Certified Neuroscience Registered Nurse
CNS	Certified Nurse Specialist
CNSD	Certified Nutrition Support Dietitian
CO	Certified Orthoptist
COA	Certified Ophthalmic Assistant
COHC	Certified Occupational Hearing Conservationist
COHN	Certified Occupational Health Nurse
COHN(C)	Certified Nurse, Critical Care, Occupational Health
COHN-S	Certified Occupational Health Nurse Specialist

COMT	Certified Ophthalmic Medical Technologist
CON(C)	Certified Nurse, Critical Care, Oncology
COT	Certified Ophthalmic Technologist
COTA	Certified Occupational Therapy Assistant
COTA/L	Certified Occupational Therapy Assistant, Licensed
CPAN	Certified PeriAnesthesia Nurse
CPFT	Certified Pulmonary Function Technologist
CPHQ	Certified Professional in Healthcare Quality
CPMHN(C)	Certified Psychiatric Mental Health Nurse
CPN	Certified Pediatric Nurse
CPN(C)	Certified Perioperative Nurse (also CNOR)
CPNP	Certified Pediatric Nurse Practitioner
CPON	Certified Pediatric Oncology Nurse
CPP	Certified Pain Practitioner
CPT	Community Practice Teacher
CPTC	Certified Procurement Transplant Coordinator
CRA	Certified Retinal Angiographer
CRC	Certified Rehabilitation Counselor
CRN	Certified Radiology Nurse
CRNA	Certified Registered Nurse Anesthetist
CRNFA	Certified Registered Nurse First Assistant
CRNH	Certified Registered Nurse Hospice
CRNI	Certified Registered Nurse of Infusion; Certified Registered Nurse, Intravenous
CRNO	Certified Registered Nurse in Ophthalmology
CRNP	Certified Registered Nurse Practitioner
CRO	Certified Radiation Oncologist
CRRN	Certified Rehabilitation Registered Nurse
CRT	Certified Radiology Technologist
CRTT	Certified Respiratory Therapy Technologist
CS	Clinical Specialist CS; Certified Specialist
CSA	Certified Surgical Assistant
CSN	Certified School Nurse
CSP	Certified Specialist in Pediatric Nutrition
CSR	Certified Specialist in Renal Nutrition
CST	Certified Surgical Technologist
CT	Cytotechnologist

CTN	Certified Transplant Nurse; Certified Transcultural Nurse
CUNP	Certified Urologic Nurse Practitioner
CUPA	Certified Urologic Physician Assistant
CURN	Certified Urologic Registered Nurse
CWCN	Certified Wound Care Nurse
CWOCN	Certified Wound, Ostomy, and Continence Nurse
DDM	Doctor of Medical Dentistry
DDS	Doctor of Dental Surgery
DNSc	Doctor of Nursing Science
DO	Doctor of Osteopathy; Doctor of Ophthalmology
DPM	Doctor of Podiatric Medicine
DPT	Physical Therapist with a Doctorate Degree in Physical Therapy
DSN	Doctor of Science in Nursing
DTR	Dietitian Technologist Registered
EDF	Emergency Department Physician
EMT–1	Emergency Medical Technologist 1
EMT-P	Emergency Medical Technician—Paramedic
EN	Enrolled Nurse
ENC(C)	Certified Nurse, Critical Care, Emergency
ET	Enterostomal Therapist
FAAN	Fellow of the American Academy of Nursing
FAAP	Fellow American Association of Pediatrics
FACC	Fellow American College of Cardiology
FACCE	Fellow in the American College of Childbirth Educators
FACCP	Fellow American College of Chest Physicians
FACP	Fellow of the American College of Pediatrics
FADA	Fellow of the American Diabetic Association
FCAP	Fellow College of American Pathologist
FNP	Family Nurse Practitioner
FRACP	Fellow Royal Australian College of Physicians
FS	Flying Surgeon
GNC(C)	Certified Nurse, Critical Care, Gerontology
GNP	Gerontological Nurse Practitioner

HHA	Home Health Aide
HNC	Holistic Nurse Certified by American Holistic Nurses Association
HT	Histologic Technologist
IBCLC	International Board Certified Lactation Consultant
ICN	Infection Control Nurse
ICP	Infection Control Practitioner
JD	Doctor of Jurisprudence; Doctor of Laws
KECHN	Kenya Enrolled Community Health Nurse
LBSW	Licensed Bachelor Social Worker
LC	Lactation Consultant
LCCE	Lamaze Certified Childbirth Educator
LCDC	Licensed Chemical Dependency Counselor
LCSW	Licensed Clinical Social Worker
LD	Licensed Dietitian
LDN	Licensed Dietitian/Nutritionist
LISW	Licensed Independent Social Worker
LMT	Licensed Massage Therapist
LNC	Legal Nurse Consultant
LP	Lecturer Practitioner
LPC	Licensed Professional Counselor
LPN	Licensed Practical Nurse
LPT	Licensed Psychiatric Technician; Licensed Physical Therapist
LPTA	Licensed Physical Therapist Assistant
LRCP	Licensed Respiratory Care Practitioner
LRCT	Licensed Respiratory Care Technician; Lab/Radiology Combined Technologist
LSW	Licensed Social Worker
LVN	Licensed Vocational Nurse
MD	Doctor of Medicine
ME	Medical Examiner
MFCC	Marriage Family and Child Counselor
MHA	Masters in Health Care Administration
MICN	Mobile Intensive Care Nurse
MLT	Medical Laboratory Technician

MN	Master of Nursing
MNEd	Master of Nursing Education
MPA	Master of Public Administration
MPH	Masters in Public Health
MPT	Physical Therapist with a Masters in Physical Therapy
MS	Master of Surgery; Master of Science; Master of Sociology; Masters in Health Science
MSA	Master of Science in Administration
MSD	Master of Surgical Dentistry
MSN	Master of Science in Nursing
MSP	Master of Psychology
MST	Therapeutic Massage Therapist
MSW	Master of Social Work; Master of Social Welfare; Medical Social Worker
MT	Medical Transcriptionist; Medical Technologist
NA	Nurse Aide (without certification)
NCC	Nationally Certified Counselor
NCPT	Nationally Certified Psychiatric Technologist
NCSN	National Certified School Nurse
ND	Doctor of Nursing; Nutritional Doctor
NEO	Neonatologist
NNP	Neonatal Nurse Practitioner
NP	Nurse Practitioner; Nurse Prescriber
NPP	Psychiatric Nurse Practitioner
OB	Obstetrics
OCN	Oncology Certified Nurse
OGNP	Obstetrical Gynecological Nurse Practitioner
ONC	Orthopedic Nurse Certified
OPA-C	Orthopedic Physician Assistant—Certified
OTR	Occupational Therapist, Registered
OTR/L	Occupational Therapist, Registered/Licensed
PA	Physician Assistant; Pathology Assistant
PA-C	Physician Assistant—Certified
PharmD	Doctor of Pharmacy
PhD	Doctor of Philosophy
PHN	Public Health Nurse

PMA	Podiatric Medical Assistant
PMH-NP	Psychiatric Mental Health Nurse Practitioner
PN	Parish Nurse
PNP	Pediatric Nurse Practitioner
PT	Physical Therapist
PTA	Physical Therapist Assistant
RCPT	Registered Cardiopulmonary Technologist
RCT	Registered Care Technologist
RD	Registered Dietitian
RDCS	Registered Diagnostic Cardiac Sonographer
RDMS	Registered Diagnostic Medical Sonographer
RGN	Registered General Nurse
RHIA	Registered Health Information Administrator (replaces RRA)
RHIT	Registered Health Information Technologist (replaces ART)
RKT	Registered Kinesiotherapist
RM	Registered Midwife
RMA	Registered Medical Assistant
RMG	Registered Mental Nurse
RMN	Registered Mental Health Nurse
RMT	Registered Massage Therapist
RN	Registered Nurse
RN BC	Registered Nurse Board Certified
RNAC	Registered Nurse Assessment Coordinator
RNC	Registered Nurse Certified
RNFA	Registered Nurse First Assistant
RNMH	Registered Nurse Mental Handicap
RNR	Registered Nurse Recruiter
RPFT	Registered Pulmonary Function Technologist
RPN	Registered Professional Nurse; Registered Practical Nurse
RPSGT	Registered Polysomnographic Technologist
RRT	Registered Respiratory Therapist; Registered Rehabilitation Specialist
RTCT	Registered Technologist Computerized Tomography
RTMRI	Registered Technologist Magnetic Resonance Imaging
RTR	Registered Technologist, Radiology
RVT	Registered Vascular Technologist

SP & PT	Specimen Procurement and Processing Technologist
SRN	State Registered Nurse
ST	Surgical Technologist; Speech Therapist
UAP	Unlicensed Assistive Personnel
WHCNP	Women's Health Care Nurse Practitioner
WHNP	Women's Health Nurse Practitioner
WOCN	Wound, Ostomy, Continence Nurse

COMMONLY USED EPONYMS

NOTE: The dictator may or may not dictate the eponym as a possessive form. Transcribe the phrase as it is dictated.

Achilles heel

Addison's disease

Alzheimer disease

Apgar score

Apley scratch maneuver

Babcock forceps

Babinski sign

Baker's cyst

Bartholin's abscess

Bell palsy

Bennett and Holman retractors

Braxton Hicks sign

Bruce protocol

Brudzinski sign

Buck fascia

Charcot joint

Codman exercises

Colles' fracture

Coombs' test

Cooper's ligament

Cornelia de Lange syndrome

Cozen sign

Crohn disease

Cushing disease

de Quervain tendinitis

DeMeester score

Down syndrome

Epstein-Barr virus

Finklestein's test

Fitz-Hugh-Curtis syndrome

Foley catheter

Fowler's position

Garre's disease

Graham Steell murmur

Graves' disease

Hallpike maneuver

Hashimoto's disease

Heaney clamp

Heberden's nodes

Homans' sign

Hunter's canal

Jobst stockings

Jones fracture

Junod boots

Kegel exercises
Kernig's sign
Kirschner rod
Kupffer cells
Kussmaul respirations

Lachman test
Le Fort fracture
Legionnaires' disease
LF fracture (I-III)
Lisfranc's fracture
Lloyd sign
Lou Gehrig's disease
Lyme disease

Marfan syndrome
McBurney's point
McMurray's test
Merchant's view
Mills sign
Mohs surgery
Moro's reflex
Moses' sign
Murphy's point

Neer 90/90
Nissen fundoplication

Osgood-Schlatter disease

Parkinson's disease
Parzett splint
Peyer's patches
Phalen's sign
Pope wick
Pott's anastomosis, scissors
Pott's fracture
Prader-Willi syndrome

Raynaud's phenomenon
Rhesus factor
Romberg's sign
Rovsing's sign

Salter fracture (I-V)
Schatzki's ring
Schilling test
Sjögren syndrome
Skene's glands
Speeds test
Spurling cervical distraction test
Stevens-Johnson syndrome

Tanner growth chart
Taylor tilt test
Tay-Sachs disease
Tinel's sign
Tourette syndrome
Treitz's ligament
Trendelenburg's position
Trousseau's sign
Tuli's heel cap
Turner sign
Tzanck smear

Valsalva maneuver

Waters view of the sinuses
Weber test
Wolfe-Parkinson-White
Wood's lamp
Wurd catheter

Zung testing

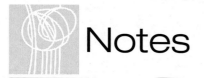

Notes

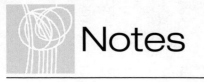

Notes

Notes

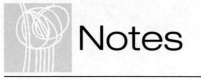

Notes

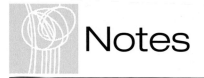

Notes

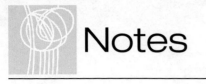

Notes

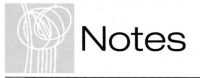 Notes

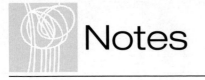

Notes

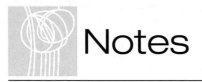

Notes

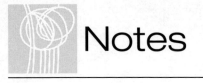

Notes

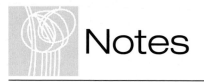

Notes

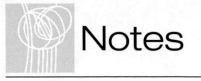

Notes

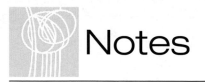

Notes

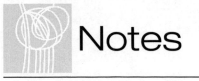 Notes